MW01600637

Keto for women over 50 + cookbook

How you can start your weight loss path using meal plans and recipes easy to cook in even less than 10 minutes

Contents

Keto after 50

Beginners guide for women over 50 to start your ketogenic diet and reset your metabolism. Included a 7-day meal plan and a special BONUS about intermittent fasting

[Jason white]

Legal & Disclaimer

The information contained in this book and its contents is not designed to replace or take the place of any form of medical or professional advice; and is not meant to replace the need for independent medical, financial, legal or other professional advice or services, as may be required. The content and information in this book have been provided for educational and entertainment purposes only.

The content and information contained in this book has been compiled from sources deemed reliable, and it is accurate to the best of the Author's knowledge, information, and belief. However, the Author cannot guarantee its accuracy and validity and cannot be held liable for any errors and/or omissions. Further, changes are periodically made to this book as and when needed. Where appropriate and/or necessary, you must consult a professional (including but not limited to your doctor, attorney, financial advisor or such other professional advisor) before using any of the suggested remedies, techniques, or information in this book.

Upon using the contents and information contained in this book, you agree to hold harmless the Author from and against any damages, costs, and expenses, including any legal fees potentially resulting from the application of any of the information provided by this book. This disclaimer applies to any loss, damages or injury caused by the use and application, whether directly or indirectly, of any advice or information presented, whether for breach of contract, tort, negligence, personal injury, criminal intent, or under any other cause of action.

You agree to accept all risks of using the information presented inside this book.

You agree that by continuing to read this book, where appropriate and/or necessary, you shall consult a professional (including but not limited to your doctor, attorney, or financial advisor or such other advisor as needed) before using any of the suggested remedies, techniques, or information in this book.

Introduction

Before starting any diet, it is crucial you understand the history behind it. As you well know, there are many diets on the market in the modern age. The right question you need to ask for yourself is, Is the Ketogenic Diet right for you? Luckily for all of us, the Ketogenic Diet can help a wide range of individuals, whether you are young, older, or somewhere in between!

History of the Ketogenic Diet

The Ketogenic Diet first began in the 1920s and 30s. Initially, it was a popular therapy for individuals who had epilepsy. At the very beginning, the Ketogenic Diet was first developed to provide an alternative to fasting, which also worked well for epilepsy therapy.

While the diet did work for a while for these patients, it was eventually abandoned when modern medicine came around and was able to help most patients with their symptoms. However, there were still approximately 30% of patients

where the medication did not work, and the diet was re-introduced to help these individuals.

In 1921, it was an endocrinologist known as Rollin Woodrat that was one of the first to notice the three water-soluble compounds that are produced in the liver when we are starved from carbohydrates. These three compounds are what we now know as ketone bodies. It was at this point, an individual from the Mayo Clinic known as Russel Wilder would call this "starvation from carbohydrates" as the Ketogenic Diet!

It is imperative to note that the ketogenic diet for people in their 30s is different from those in their 50s. The main difference is in the amount of energy required to do various activities. In your younger years, you will need more energy to allow you to carry out your activities easily. There is solid evidence that a ketogenic diet can reduced seizures. Since it has neuroprotective features, your brain cells will be replenished, and you will not experience memory loss quickly. Some studies suggest that a ketogenic diet can help in preventing disorders such as Alzheimer's, sleep disorders, autism, and Parkinson's disease. Weight loss is the most important aspect of a ketogenic diet, and you can easily lose weight with the ketogenic diet. It will help in improving blood sugar levels as well as rejuvenating your brain cells as well as give you a feel-good mood.

Although the diet is solely based on fats and proteins, you should try and take fats and proteins that are healthy. Avoid processed salty foods as well as fats with low-density lipoproteins. Eating healthy is the first way of building a better immune system and a better mood throughout the day. Choose the ketogenic diet and enjoy the benefits that come with it.

Most of the sugar that we consume is a pure form of glucose; on the other hand, some of the carbohydrates can be broken down into glucose. When the body runs low on glucose, it can break down fats into energy, and this is a process called gluconeogenesis. Besides, the body can run on other energy sources such as free fatty acids and ketones. However, it is important to note that the body will only run on alternative sources of energy once glucose is depleted in the system. The depletion of glucose in the body usually results from fasting or eating a diet that is low in carbohydrates.

The glucose depletion process can take anywhere from 24 to 36 hours, although this process can be sped up by carrying out various forms of exercises. As the glucose reserves get depleted, the body will compensate for the energy needs by burning free fatty acids.

As the diet continues to grow in popularity, there is more research being performed on the Ketogenic Diet by the day! With science backed evidence, you can follow the diet and know for a fact that it is going to work.

Welcome to your first Ketogenic Diet Science lesson! One of the best parts of the Ketogenic Diet is the fact that it is based around a natural process that your body already has! The key to success is fueling your body correctly instead of stuffing it with overly processed junk. In this guide, you will learn everything you need to know from what to eat when to eat and how to get into the best shape of your life!

Chapter 1: What is Keto Diet

The Ketogenic Diet follows a simple principle: keep your food consumption low-carb and high-fat. So basically, being on the diet means eating less carbohydrates and adding more fats in your daily meals. Do not be confused. When we say "fat" we are not talking about the literal kind that is attached to your body. Fat has gotten a bad reputation nowadays, but "fat" the nutrient is actually very different from the "fat" that makes your clothes fit tight.

Good fats are the kind you get from avocado, nuts, and fish. For example, there are the omega-3 and omega-6 fatty acids that help you lose weight, get better heart health, and have excellent hair and nails.

Why Do People Lose Weight on the Keto Diet and Get Healthier?

Naturally, the question that is asked about the Keto Diet is why so many of your friends who are on the Keto Diet seem to be losing so much weight so quickly. The reality is that in the first three to six months on the Keto diet, the body is dropping a tremendous amount of weight because of how the diet is forcing the body to draw energy. Remember how it was said earlier how the body likes to use blood sugar because blood sugar is an easy way to draw energy without using too much energy? Well, what happens when the blood sugar is not in large supply?

This is the essence of the weight loss with the Keto Diet. The reality is that weight loss occurs because it takes a lot of calories to burn a single fat cell compared to the calories needed to use blood sugar. The same is true for the protein that is in the body. There is also a psychological element at play here. Carbs can be empty calories and they are really easy to convert into energy – in fact, as you are chewing a piece of bread the body is getting the nutrients from it, whereas if you are eating something that is denser – like meat – then what happens is the digestion occurs in the stomach. It takes much energy to digest a high fat, high protein diet. And – here is the good news – who does not like to have a diet where they can eat things that they love?! This is the great part about the Keto Diet. The high fat and high protein that goes into the diet provides what the body needs in calories to fire up the burning of the fat cells that are critical to losing weight.

The other reason why people lose weight on this diet is because there is less production of insulin by the body. The insulin is used up quickly, and the body does not need as much on the Keto Diet. Insulin is made by the body in response to excessive carbohydrates. They are the fuel needed to build insulin. Insulin gets stored in the body because it is essential to storing sugar as fuel. The sugar getting stored in the body is gradually eliminated through the Keto Diet. So, with less insulin that means there is less sugar your body is storing. And another ancillary benefit of this is there is a connection between less insulin in the body and instances of cancer.

Besides cancer and insulin issues, one thing that the Keto Diet has a massive effect on is cholesterol. The difference between HDL and LDL is simple – LDL is the bad cholesterol that clogs the arteries and restricts blood flow. This is the cholesterol that builds the arterial plaque that ends up killing people at worst and if it is found, it is the stuff that leads to having stents and pacemakers put into people's hearts. The reality is the more LDL in a person, the worse off they are with their heart. That is why the Keto Diet seems to be counterintuitive – this is a diet that is telling you to eat more fat. But here is the thing, there are two types of fats – good fats and bad fats. Now, here is how the Keto Diet affects your cholesterol production. The key to production of cholesterol is levels of insulin. The more insulin that is stored in your body, the more you will have to deal with cholesterol being something that affects you. In fact, when you use the Keto Diet, what will happen is that your levels of cholesterol will decrease because there is not enough insulin to make the cholesterol. When there is less cholesterol in your system, this means the chances of your arteries hardening and there being blockages that could lead to heart failure lessen as well.

For seniors, this is especially important because cardiovascular health is one of the keys to a good long life. The Keto Diet provides seniors with an easy way to maintain their heart health. So, whether they are people who have had heart issues in the past or are looking to make sure they do not have heart issues in the future, the Keto Diet is a great way to keep them healthy, especially in terms of their heart and the other parts of the cardiovascular system. The less cholesterol the better, and if it means that the diet keeps them from having to take statins to reduce cholesterol, that is all the better.

Another issue that affects seniors disproportionately is diabetes. The problem with diabetes is that essentially the blood sugar in your system is way too high, and this messes with insulin and a whole host of other problems. So, when you are on a low carb diet such as the Keto Diet, then what happens is your blood sugar lowers. The lowering of your blood sugar occurs because the body is not creating as much blood sugar as it burns. When you start to burn fat, this produces greater amounts of ketones in your blood stream. However, for people with Type 1 Diabetes, you do not want to have too many ketones in your blood stream. Therefore, it is vitally important that you check with your doctor. For people looking to prevent Type 2 diabetes, making sure that you are limiting your intake of carbs is the simple way to make sure that you are not having to deal with the effects of having too much insulin. That is why it is imperative if you use the Keto Diet to implement it fully. For seniors, this is a great way to avoid having to do the finger pricks and insulin injections.

Other reasons that seniors may want to try the Keto Diet have to do with nervous system disorders that often come about during their elderly years, specifically Alzheimer's and Parkinson's. These disorders are primarily located in the brain and have to do with the degradation of brain cells. The key is protecting the brain cells, and nutrition plays a part in it. There has been a lot scientific research into the effects that ketones have on people who are elderly, and one thing that researchers have found is that ketones act as a bit of a shield for Parkinson's and for Alzheimer's. These are disorders that profoundly affect the quality of life that seniors have, so therefore it is imperative that seniors make sure that they are having a good diet that promotes the larger numbers of ketones in the body. Doing so will ensure that blood sugar stays low, and when blood sugar is low, this means that the guardians to the brain cells are that much more fortified. When the brain cells are processing tasks efficiently and not getting bogged down with insulin, this has some real effects ho the way that people can remain healthy in a cognitive way for the remainder of their years, especially when considering the crippling way that Alzheimer's and Parkinson's have in terms of quality of life and to financial health.

For active seniors, the Keto Diet is great, so for people who still like to get in their walks or their bike rides, it is imperative to make sure that they are having a diet that is rich in protein and in good fats. This helps the body process the protein and the endurance athletes especially appreciate it because it allows them to compete and move for extended periods of time without cramping or dealing with muscular fatigue that could impact performance. In fact, having a good muscle to fat ratio is imperative for efficiently using oxygen in the blood stream, so this is something that is important. If a senior is looking to stick with bike riding and other sports like this, it is a good idea to be on the Keto Diet because this diet promotes the important things that help them stay with their training and have the best possible performance under a variety of circumstances.

Chapter 2: How Keto Diet works after age 50

What Happens to Your Body When You Eat Keto?

Even before we talk about how to do keto – it is important to first consider why this diet works. What happens to your body to make you lose weight?

As you probably know, the body uses food as an energy source. Everything you eat is turned into energy, so that you can get up and do whatever you need to accomplish for the day. The main energy source is sugar so what happens is that you eat something, the body breaks it down into sugar, and the sugar is processed into energy. Typically, the "sugar" is taken directly from the food you eat so if you eat just the right amount of food, then your body is fueled for the whole day. If you eat too much, then the sugar is stored in your body – hence the accumulation of fat.

But what happens if you eat less food? This is where the Ketogenic Diet comes in. You see, the process of creating sugar from food is usually faster if the food happens to be rich in carbohydrates. Bread, rice, grain, pasta – all of these are carbohydrates and they are the easiest food types to turn into energy.

So, the Ketogenic Diet is all about reducing the amount of carbohydrates you eat. Does this mean you will not get the kind of energy you need for the day? Of course not! It only means that now, your body must find other possible sources of energy. Do you know where they will be getting that energy? Your stored body fat!

So, here is the situation – you are eating less carbohydrates every day. To keep you energetic, the body breaks down the stored fat and turns them into molecules called ketone bodies. The process of turning the fat into ketone bodies is called "Ketosis" and obviously – this is where the name of the Ketogenic Diet comes from. The ketone bodies take the place of glucose in keeping you energetic. If you keep your carbohydrates reduced, the body will keep getting its energy from your body fat.

Sounds Simple, Right?

The Ketogenic Diet is often praised for its simplicity and when you look at it properly, the process is straightforward. The Science behind the effectivity of the diet is also well-documented and has been proven multiple times by different medical fields. For example, an article on Diet Review by Harvard provided a lengthy discussion on how the Ketogenic Diet works and why it is so effective for those who choose to use this diet.

But Fat Is the Enemy...Or Is It?

No – fat is NOT the enemy. Unfortunately, years of bad science told us that fat is something you must avoid – but it is actually an extremely helpful thing for weight loss! Even before we move forward with this book, we will have to discuss exactly what "healthy fats" are, and why they are the good guys. To do this, we need to make a distinction between the different kinds of fat. You have probably heard of them before and it is a little bit confusing at first. We will try to go through them as simply as possible:

Saturated fat. This is the kind you want to avoid. They are also called "solid fat" because each molecule is packed with hydrogen atoms. Simply put, it is the kind of fat that can easily cause a blockage in your body. It can raise cholesterol levels and lead to heart problems or a stroke. Saturated fat is something you can find in meat, dairy products, and other processed food items. Now, you are probably wondering: isn't the Ketogenic Diet packed with saturated fat? The answer is: not necessarily. You will find later in the recipes given that the Ketogenic Diet promotes primarily unsaturated fat or healthy fat. While there are many meat recipes in the list, most of these recipes contain healthy fat sources.

Unsaturated Fat. These are the ones dubbed as healthy fat. They are the kind of fat you find in avocado, nuts, and other ingredients you usually find in Keto-friendly recipes. They are known to lower blood cholesterol and come in two types: polyunsaturated and monounsaturated. Both are good for your body, but the benefits slightly vary, depending on what you are consuming.

Polyunsaturated fat. These are perhaps the best in the list. You know about omega-3 fatty acids, right? They are often suggested for people who have heart problems and are recognized as the "healthy" kind of fat. Well, they fall under the category of polyunsaturated fat and are known for reducing risks of heart disease by as much as 19 percent. This is according to a study titled: Effects on coronary heart diseases of increased poly-unsaturated fat in lieu of saturated fat: systematic review & meta-analysis of randomized controlled tests. So where do you get these polyunsaturated fats? You can get them mostly from vegetable and seed oils. These are ingredients you can almost always find in Ketogenic Recipes such as olive oil, coconut oil, and more. If you need more convincing, you should also know that omega-3 fatty acids are a kind of polyunsaturated fats and you will find them in deep sea fish like tuna, herring, and salmon.

How keto diets works for weight loss

Ketogenic diet works by forcing the body to enter a state called ketosis. The body usually uses carbohydrate as its primary energy source. This is because the carbohydrates are the easiest to absorb for the body.

If the body runs out of carbohydrates, however, it will revert to making use of fats and protein to produce energy. The body has a kind of hierarchy of energy that follows.

First, when available, the body is programmed to use carbohydrate as a fuel for energy. Second, in the absence of adequate carbohydrate supply, it will return to the use of fats as an alternative.

Finally, when its carbohydrate and fat stores are extremely depleted, the body will turn to protein for its energy supply. Breakdown of proteins for energy supply, however, results in a general loss of lean muscle mass. The keto diet does not depend entirely on the calories in, calories out model. This is because, due to the body's hormonal response to different macronutrients, the composition of these calories matters.

In the keto community, though, there are two schools of thought. While one believes that calories and fat consumption are irrelevant, the other argues that calories and fat are important.

You are trying to find a balance point when using a keto diet. While calories matter, it also counts the composition of those calories. The most important factor in the composition of these calories in a keto diet is the balance of fat, protein, and carbohydrates and how each affects the levels of insulin.

Because any increase in insulin will stop lipolysis, this balance is especially important. You therefore need to eat foods that create the smallest increase in insulin. This will help keep your body in the fuel-lipolysis state of burning stored body fat.

Normally, the body can go alone into a ketosis state. This often happens when you are in a state of fasting, like when you are sleeping. In this state, while the body repairs and grows while you sleep, the body tends to burn fats for energy.

Carbohydrates in a regular meal generally make up most of the calories. Also, as it is easier to absorb, the body is inclined to use the carbohydrate as energy. Therefore, the diet's proteins and fats are more likely to be stored.

However, most calories are derived from fats rather than carbohydrates in a keto diet. Because keto diets have low carbohydrate levels, they are used up immediately. The low level of carbohydrate causes the body's apparent lack of energy fuel.

The body resorts to its stored fat content because of this apparent shortage. It makes a shift from a consumer of carbohydrate to a fat burner. However, in the recently ingested meal, the body does not use the fats, but instead stores them for the next round of ketosis.

As the body becomes more familiar with burning fat for energy, fats are used up for storage in an ingested meal with little left.

That is why the keto diet uses a high amount of fat intake so that the body can have enough to produce energy and store some fat. The body must be able to store some fat otherwise during the ketosis period it will begin to break down its protein stores in the muscles.

The body still needs a constant supply of energy during fasting periods- such as during ketosis, between meals and during sleep. You have these times in your normal day, so you need to consume enough fat to use your body as energy.

If there are no adequate quantities of stored fat, your muscle's proteins will be the next option for the body to use as energy. Therefore, it is important to eat enough to avoid this scenario.

A keto diet's main goal is to mimic the body's hunger state. By restricting and severely reducing the intake of carbohydrates, keto diets deprive the body of its preferred immediate and easily convertible carbohydrates. This situation forces it into a mode of fat burning to produce energy.

Chapter 3: Benefits of Keto Diet after age 50

People who engage in Keto diet, particularly those aged 50 and older, are said to reap various potential health benefits including:

Improved physical and mental strength

When people grow older, energy levels that fall for a variety of biological and environmental reasons. Adherents to the Keto diet often experience a boost in strength and vitality. One reason the occurrence is because the body burns excess fat, which is synthesized into energy in turn.

Metabolism

Aging people often experience a slower metabolism than they have experienced in their younger days. Long-term keto dieters undergo increased blood glucose control, which may improve their metabolic rates.

Protection against specific diseases

Keto dieters over 50 years of age may reduce their risk of developing diseases such as diabetes, mental disorders such as Alzheimer's, various cardiovascular diseases, various types of cancer, Parkinson's disease, non-alcoholic fatty liver disease (NAFLD) and multiple sclerosis.

Some consider aging to be the most important risk factor for human disease or illness. Reducing ageing is therefore a logical step towards reducing these disease risk factors.

Good news from the technical description of the ketosis cycle mentioned earlier, reveals the increased energy of the youth as a consequence and because of the use of fat as a source of fuel, the body can go through a phase where signals can be misinterpreted so that the mTOR signal is blocked and a loss of insulin is apparent where ageing is stated to be slowed down.

Multiple studies have commonly recognized for years that caloric restriction can help slow the aging process and even increasing the lifespan. With the ketogenic diet, it is important to influence anti-aging without increasing calories. The periodic form of fasting used with the keto diet may also impact vascular ageing.

When a human fast intermittently or is developed on a keto diet, it is suspected that BHB or Beta-Hydroxybutyrate causes anti-aging results.

Quite small in carbs and typically strong in fats and/or proteins, ketogenic diets are used successfully for weight loss during overweight and heart disease care. However, an important note in the article was that "Results on the impact of such diets on cardiovascular risk factors are controversial" and "In addition, these diets are not completely safe and may be associated with some adverse events. More is required than merely researching this diet, advantages, positive effects, and side effects, particularly in aged adults on the Internet. One should speak to his or her medical professional about specific concerns.

Chapter 4: Keto Diet Plan for 50+ aged people

Step 1

Calculate and track your macros. Macronutrients (macros) are carbohydrates, fats, and proteins. An average person would need more fat and fewer carbs, while a professional athlete may need more protein and high carbohydrate consumption.

Track your calorie consumption. Skipping a meal here or there is not harmful when it is occasional but restricting calories for longer periods can have negative effects on your health. Carb cycling also involves calorie cycling so you can switch from low-calorie to higher-calorie periods.

Keep an eye on the amount of cholesterol. If your cholesterol level is high, avoid saturated fats (found primarily in red meat) and opt for monounsaturated fats. Trans fats such as partially hydrogenated vegetable oils are out of the question; they can be found in margarine and other spreads, fried foods, packaged foods, and fast foods. On the other hand, you should increase soluble fiber, foods rich in omega-3 fatty acid (herring, salmon, mackerel, flaxseeds, and walnuts).

Replenish electrolytes. Just make sure that you are eating foods that contain electrolytes such as bouillon, leafy green, avocado, and Himalayan salt. Taking magnesium supplements may be beneficial on a keto diet.

A few more tips. Consume at least 8 glasses of water per day to stay hydrated on the ketogenic diet. Further, get regular exercise. It does not have to be anything special and time-consuming. Simply find an activity that fits into your schedule like walking, cycling, or stair climbing. Keep it simple since the ketogenic diet requires a little pre-planning. Stick to real and nutrient-dense foods and find good alternatives for your favorite carbs. I am sure you will find inspiration and motivation in these six hundred recipes. You will learn how to prepare keto pancakes, granola, desserts, waffles, and snacks. It is all about variety and smart food choices, not rigid rules, and restrictive diet plans. And remember – you are beautiful just the way you are, take a deep breath and love yourself.

Weigh Your Food: Being accurate about your macros is very crucial to the success of the ketogenic diet. Make sure that invest in a good food scale so that you can monitor your macro intake. So, avoid the guesswork and use a scale to measure your food. If you have more money to spare, buy scales that you can connect to apps and websites.

• **Drink Water:** Staying hydrated is one of the most important rules when it comes to following any kinds of diet regimen. Start your day by consuming at least 8 to 16 ounces of water to allow the body to begin its natural cycle.

• **Exercise:** Remember that diet alone will not help you lose as much weight as you want. You can also do resistant training because it requires more protein to aid in muscle gain. This exercise is great for keeping your protein in check especially if you consumed more of it than fats. Make sure that you match this diet regimen with a high interval and high-intensity workout to improve your blood glucose levels. Exercise at least 25 minutes every day to see the best results.

• **Reduce Your Stress:** Stress can affect your hormone levels by causing your blood sugar level to rise thus increasing your cravings. Have you ever noticed why you often crave for sweets when you are stressed out? That is your hormone talking. While you cannot control the stress that comes your way, find ways on how to mitigate it. You can practice yoga, mindfulness, and breathing exercises to take away your stress.

• **Choose Quality Carbs:** Some of you may say that carb is carb no matter what form they exist in. But remember that not all carbs are created equally. There are carbs that are nutrient-rich and are found in non-starchy vegetables and some fruits. So, when making a meal plan, make sure that you use good quality carbs.

- **Stay Away from Diet Soda:** Just because it comes with the word "diet" with it does not mean that it is good for you. Diet soda uses a wide variety of sugar substitutes that tells your body that is has an overload of sugar thereby shutting the metabolism down. So, if you need to quench your thirst, drink sparkling water instead.

- **Get Enough Sleep:** Sleep is necessary for you to lose weight fast. Remember that the lack of sleep causes stress to the body. Stress, as I have discussed earlier can affect the hormone levels in your body thus increasing your cravings to constantly snack on food. So, make sure that you get at least 6 to 8 hours of sleep daily.

- **Intermittent Fasting:** If you genuinely want to lose weight fast with the ketogenic diet, you might want to consider pairing it with intermittent fasting. Intermittent fasting is when you fast for more than 12 hours so that your body will use up the stored fats as its primary fuel. Consume your keto-friendly meals within a short eating window time and the rest of the day should be dedicated to no food consumption so that your body can undergo the state of ketosis faster. For instance, you can go fasting from 2:00 pm to 8:00 am the following day. From 8:01 am to 1:59 pm, that is the only time you allow yourself to eat your meals.

Step 2

You must remember that just like all other diet regimens, not everyone can follow a ketogenic diet. So, before you start this regimen, ask yourself if the ketogenic diet is really for you? Below are the things that you should consider seeing if the ketogenic diet is for you.

- **How long can I follow this diet?** The ketogenic diet is not like your usual fad diet only lasting for a few weeks. To see results, it will take you months or even a year. So, if you are someone who cannot follow its principles long-term, then this diet is not for you.

- **Will the eating plan fit my food preference, budget needs, and culture?** If you follow a strict dietary guideline (veganism or vegetarianism) then you might need to tweak the ketogenic diet to fit your preferences. It may difficult, but not impossible. However, if you find it too much of a hassle to tweak the ketogenic meal plan to fit your preference, you might not enjoy this diet at all.

• **Do I have medical conditions that will put me at risk?** While the ketogenic diet has therapeutic effects to people who suffer from diabetes and cardiovascular diseases, it is not prescribed among people who suffer from kidney-related problems as the presence of protein and fats can be damaging to the kidneys.

The bottom line is that while the ketogenic diet is good for most people, it may not be advisable for some. So, before you ask yourself if this diet is for you, make sure that you seek advice from your nutritionist or physician.

Since the carbohydrate intake for this diet is kept at an exceptionally low, carbs are practically absent thus the body is pushed to utilize other forms of energy in the form of fat.

In the absence of fat, the liver takes the fatty acids in the body then converts it into ketone bodies. You must remember that the body just cannot take fat and use it in its raw form. It must undergo different processes so that it can be utilized effectively by the body. This is the reason why it needs to convert it into ketone form. This process is called ketosis, and this is what the ketogenic diet is all about.

In a nutshell, there are three types of ketone bodies created during the break down of fatty acids and these include (1) acetoacetate, (2) beta-hydroxybutyric acid, and (3) acetone.

There are numerous benefits of the keto diet aside from weight loss and better energy levels.

• **Better blood sugar control:** The ketogenic diet lowers the blood sugar levels thus making it a great way to manage or even prevent diabetes. The thing is that the body takes a rest from producing insulin thus it can stabilize itself during ketosis.

• **Improved mental focus:** Several studies suggest that the ketogenic diet can increase health performance. Because this diet does not spike blood sugar levels, the brain is kept in a stable condition. Moreover, the brain simply loves ketones as its primary source of fuel.

• **Reduced cravings and hunger pains:** Fats are known to be filling, so this diet does not only curb your cravings but also reduces hunger pains.

• **Better cholesterol and blood pressure levels:** This diet regimen can improve triglyceride and cholesterol levels in the body. This reduces the risk of developing clogged arteries.

• **Clearer skin:** Didn't you know that the ketogenic diet can help improve the quality of your skin? Several studies suggest that people who follow the ketogenic diet often experience clearing of their acne and other skin anomalies. The ketogenic diet, aside from pushing ketosis, also drives the immune system into a frenzy thus it can help eliminate inflammation on the skin.

Before you can experience the many benefits of the ketogenic diet, it is important that you eat mostly fat. But how much fat is too much? When I first started, I had this misinformed idea that all I need to do is to eat all the fatty foods that I see. This was easy as pie, I said. And to tell you the truth, I see countless of dieters out there who make the same mistake that I did.

To succeed with the ketogenic diet, you do not need to eat a lot of fat. Rather, you need to smartly break down what you eat to 70-80% fat, 20-25% protein, and 5-10% carbohydrates.

You must remember that the ratio varies depending on different people thus using an online calculator can greatly help! Make sure that you stick by your macros. The problem with most people is that they tend to eat more protein thinking that protein is always equivalent to fat. Well, not quite. Once you consume protein, the protein will be broken down into a process known as gluconeogenesis and it converts protein into carbs. So, you are back to square one.

To ensure that your body is constantly in the state of ketosis, you need to test the ketone levels in your body to know whether your body is still driving under this state or if you reverted back to your usual glucose-feeding metabolism.

There are several ways to test your body for the presence of ketones. Remember that when your body starts to burn off fats as its main energy source, ketones are spilled over into your blood and urine. And it is even present in you breathe! Since ketones are spilled all over the body, you can test either your urine or breath for its presence. You do not need to punch a tiny hole on your skin for blood testing.

Chapter 5: What to Eat and What to Avoid during Keto Diet

What Can You Eat When You Are over 50?

As we know that the ketogenic diet is low carb high fat and an adequate amount of protein diet. The following is the food list that allows during the keto diet.

Fats: Fat is necessary during keto diet because near about 75 to 90percent of calories come from fat.

Oils: Instead of processed oil, use oils come from seeds and nuts some keto-friendly oils are coconut oil, butter, avocado oil, MCT oils, lard, extra virgin olive oil, and macadamia oils.

Nuts and seeds: Nuts and seeds are one of the best choices during keto diet because it is high in fat and low in carb. Some keto-friendly nuts and seeds are brazil nuts, pecans, hazelnuts, walnuts, macadamia nuts, pumpkin seeds, flaxseeds, chia seeds, sesame seeds, almonds, and hemp seeds.

Proteins: Adequate amount of proteins (5 to 20 %) are needed during the ketogenic diet.

Meat: Organic and grass-fed meats prefer during the keto diet. Unprocessed meats are low in carb and high in protein. Beef, pork, wild game, veal, and lamb are the best choices for the keto diet.

Poultry: Chicken, Cornish hen, pheasant, quails, duck, turkey, and eggs are the best choices during the keto diet.

Seafood: Salmon, cod, catfish, mahi-mahi, halibut, tuna, trout, octopus, oyster, clams, and shellfish are the best choice during the keto diet.

Dairy: Use high-fat dairy products instead of low fat because the low-fat dairy product contains added sugar. Heavy cream, butter, yogurt, parmesan cheese, cheddar cheese, feta cheese, Colby cheese, mascarpone, Swiss cheese, and mozzarella is the healthy choice during the keto diet.

Carbohydrates: Keto diet is a low carb diet it requires 5 percent of calories from carb intake.

Fruits: Low calories fruits are preferred during the keto diet. Avocado, lemon, blackberries, raspberries, watermelon, and strawberry are the best choices during the keto diet.

Vegetables: Green and leafy vegetables are one of the healthiest choices during keto diet because they are low in carb and high in nutrients. Spinach, chives, asparagus, radicchio, broccoli, cabbage, Brussels sprout, zucchini, celery, chard, bell peppers, olives, etc.

Drinks: During keto diet drink plenty of water to keep your body hydrated. You can also drink plain water, coconut milk, lemon water, almond milk, and low-carb juices.

Condiments: Condiments are used for flavor, you can use low-carb marinara sauce, soy sauce, unsweetened ketchup, yellow mustard all these condiments are no added sugar.

What You Can't Eat When You Are over 50?

Here is a list of foods that should avoid during ketogenic diet

Fats to avoid

Avoid refined oils they contain omega-6 fatty acids which raise your blood pressure. Soybean oil, sunflower oil, peanut oil, corn oil, sesame oil, margarine, grape-seed oil. Also, avoid packed foods that contain processed Trans fats.

Protein to avoid

Avoid processed meats, packed sausage, canned meat, smoked meat, beef jerky, hotdogs, fatless cheese, sweetened yogurt, salami.

Carb to avoid

Avoid starchy vegetables like potato, parsnip, beets, yucca, corn, peas, and sweet potato these vegetables are high in carb.

Avoid Fruits like mango, pear, dates, raisins, grapes, pineapple, apple are high in carb and sugar.

Avoid legumes and beans like black beans, kidney beans, fava beans, lima beans, chickpeas, pinto beans, oatmeal, lentils, and cereals. It contains high-carb values.

Avoid whole grains like wheat, rice, bulgur, quinoa, oat, barley, and buckwheat.

Sweeteners to avoid

Avoid maple syrup, agave nectar, honey, sugar, corn syrup, sucralose, and Splenda.

Drinks to avoid

During keto diet avoid sweetened and processed drinks like tea, coffee, soda, sugar, milk, and fruit juices. Avoid Alcohol like liquor, beer, sweetened cocktail, and wine. It is also responsible to rise in blood sugar.

Chapter 6: Common mistakes in following Keto Diet for people above age 50

There is no point in starting a lifestyle changing diet if you do not follow the guidelines properly. Here are a few common mistakes you should avoid when you are starting keto:

Not Getting Enough Shuteye As we have mentioned before, the keto diet is a significant lifestyle change. Allow your body to relax and refuel. Your body requires adequate sleep to support quick metabolism. Plus, when you are tired and groggy all day, you are likely to opt for snacks to keep yourself energized. We highly suggest you get between seven to nine hours of sleep every day. Sneaking an afternoon nap will also do wonders for you.

Not Going to A Doctor and Going It Alone

You have read up on all the benefits of keto on the internet and you are eager to get started... but wait. Before you dive into the world of low-card meal plans, consider visiting your doctor to talk about your dietary needs. As healthy as this book is, your doctor should be onboard, especially if you are taking medication. Depending on your health, the doctors may prescribe alternate medication to match your new lifestyle. For instance, your doctor may recommend a lower dose of insulin now that you are already limiting carbs in your diet. Also, have you ever had a gym buddy? Well, getting yourself a keto buddy will also do you some good. Try starting Keto with your partner or with a close friend. Having a buddy will serve as a continued source of motivation for you.

Hoarding onto Snacks Snacks are a great way to keep yourself energized throughout the day but hoarding onto cheese and nuts will not do you well. These snacks will sneak in more calories to your diet. Only use snacks as way to end hunger during meals. It is easier to fall that excessive snacking path. Other than that, give your body time to utilize stored fat for energy.

Not Preparing Yourself for The Keto Flu

Once your body starts depleting fats, you may start to experience certain flu like symptoms. This includes nausea, fatigue, aches, and cramps. If you have not looked up the symptoms or have not prepared to tackle these symptoms in advance, you may feel the need to give up the diet completely.

Also, since you are likely to be low on energy the following days, we suggest your meal prep in advance. Going thorough dietary changes can be daunting hence we advise that you start taking it easy. One other way to minimize the impact of the Keto Flu is to add more potassium and sodium in your diet.

Adding Too Much Dairy in Your Diet For many folks, cheese can have a counter effect on your diet and may prevent you from losing weight. Cheese is high in proteins and can also prevent weight loss. This is because dairy foods are a combination of proteins, fats, and carbs.

So yes, while cheese may technically be a keto friendly snack, do not consume too much. Moderation is the key, so keep it to about 1 or 2 ounces of cheese or cream per meal.

Not Consuming Enough Omega-3 Fatty Acids

While fat is the hero of this diet, do not use it as a field day for stocking up on creamy cheeses and bacon. Add healthy fats to your diet, particularly those that contain omega-3 fatty acids. These healthy fats are typically found in foods such as muscles, oysters, sardines, and salmon. Avocados and flaxseed are also forming of healthy fats since they contain monounsaturated and polyunsaturated fats that are good for you.

Consuming healthy fats will help you in feeling full, and it might just do some good to your hair, skin, and nails.

Not Being Watchful of Your Stress Levels

As you approach your 50s, we realize that a lot of stress can kick in. But being healthy, calm, and relaxed is important. Chronic stress can have a significant negative impact on your body. For instance, high levels of cortisol (a stress hormone) can increase your chances of gaining weight.

Therefore, we advise you take up a self-relieving activity to complement your diet.

Doing yoga, light exercises are some simple ways to keep you calm. If matters get worse, you can seek help from a professional or even take up mediation. Being healthy is not just about eating the right foods, it also about feeding your soul and mind with happy thoughts.

Chapter 7: Shopping list

Chapter 3: What to Eat and What to Avoid

What to Eat on Keto?

Ketones form when a person follows a low carb/high protein diet. Once the body enters Ketosis, the liver uses the fat to produce the Ketones. The production of Ketones helps improve blood flow to the brain resulting in quicker thinking and improved concentration. This makes the Keto diet great for women who are struggling with brain fog during menopause and post menopause.

The Keto diet suggests typically a limit of 20 to 50 grams of carbohydrates per day. While this can seem like a challenge, there are so many other food alternatives. Eating Keto-friendly meals never have to be boring or bland.

Seafood

Shellfish and fish are fantastic Keto diet options, they are extremely low carb and fully of healthy vitamins. Salmon and other types of fish are extremely high in B vitamins, selenium, and potassium.

You will still want to make sure that you are checking the nutritional information to ensure your carb intake doesn't go over the recommended amount.

Here is a list of seafood and the carb content based on a weight of 3.5 ounces.

- Mussels — 7 grams
- Clams — 5 grams
- Oysters — 4 grams
- Octopus — 4 grams
- Squid — 3 grams

Sardines, salmon, mackerel, and other types of fatty fish are incredibly high in omega 3, which has been found to lower the insulin levels, as well as increase sensitivity to insulin in those who are obese. Also, frequently eating fish has also been linked to improving mental health, including depression and mood swings. We suggest eating two servings of seafood weekly while on your Keto diet.

Vegetables that are low in carbs and starch are another great staple of the Keto diet. Veggies are high in nutrients and essential minerals. They are also a great source of fiber, which we all need in our diet. Vegetables also include antioxidants that aid in protection against free radicals that can cause aging.

If you are looking for ways to eat your typical foods while being on the Keto diet, then you will be surprised at what you can do. For instance, cauliflower can be cooked and mimic mashed potatoes, as well as rice. You are even able to make spaghetti noodles out of zucchini.

Cheeses

Cheese is another tasty and nutritious option while on Keto! Who does not love a great cheese board and a glass of red wine? Fortunately, all types of cheese are low in carbohydrates and high in fat content. This makes cheese perfect for the Keto diet. For example, just one ounce of cheddar cheese offers only 1 gram of carbohydrates, the protein content is 7 grams, and there is a 20 percent of RDI of calcium.

Cheese is extremely high in saturated fat; however, it has not been proven to increase heart disease risks. Some studies show that cheese can help against this risk. It also has conjugated linoleic acid. This is a type of fat that is causally linked to weight loss and has also been shown to help the body composition.

Eating cheese regularly will also help the reduction in the loss of your muscle mass, as well as strength when aging is an issue. A 12-week study showed that adults over the age of 50 that ate 7 ounces of ricotta cheese daily had an increase in their muscle mass, as well as muscle strength.

Avocados

Avocados are another great choice! In 3.5 ounces of avocados, about half of an avocado contains 9 grams of carbohydrates. However, 7 of the rams are fiber. This means that the net amount of carbs is 2 grams.

Avocados are incredibly high in many minerals and vitamins. This also includes potassium, a very crucial mineral that many women over the age of 50 are deficient in. A higher level of potassium intake will help make your transition into this diet much easier. Potassium also helps lower the frequency of muscle cramps.

In one study, people who consumed a specially designed diet that included many avocados showed positive changes in their cholesterol. Members experienced a decrease in LDL cholesterol level by 22 percent, as well as triglycerides. They also had an increase in HDL cholesterol by 11 percent.

Poultry and Meat

Poultry and meat are staple foods of almost every diet. Fresh meats and poultry include no carbohydrates and are high in B vitamins. They also contain many different minerals, including zinc, potassium, and selenium.

A study conducted with women over 50 on fatty versus non-fatty meant found that eating a diet in high-fat types of meat increase HDL cholesterol levels by 8% compared to those that ate a low level of fatty meats. It is suggested to only choose to grass-fed meat. That is due to grass-fed animals having more omega-three fats, antioxidants, and linoleum acid.

Eggs are very versatile and are one of the top healthiest foods available. One larger sized egg contains one gram of carbs and less than six grams of protein. This makes eggs an ideal food for someone on the Keto diet.

Eggs are also known to have trigger hormones that will increase the feeling of being full and will keep your blood sugar stable. This will lead to a lower number of calories consumed in 24 hours. It is essential to consume the whole egg. Most of the nutrients in an egg is found inside of the yolk. It includes zeaxanthin, which aids in the protection of eye health. It also offers a decent number of antioxidants.

Even though the yolks have a high level of cholesterol, eating eggs does not raise your blood cholesterol levels. This great food shows that it modifies the shape of your LDL and reduces heart disease risks.

Coconut Oil

Coconut oil is unique because it is exceptionally great for those who are on the Keto diet. This product includes medium-chain triglycerides. Unlike long-chain fats, MCTs are absorbed directly by your liver, and then converted into the Ketones or even used as a fast energy resource.

Coconut oil has been utilized to increase the body's Ketone levels in those with Alzheimer's disease, as well as other types of disorders of the nervous system and the brain. The primary fatty type of acid that is in coconut oil is a longer chain fat. It is called lauric acid. It is suggested that the mix of MCTs and lauric acid promotes a constant level of Ketosis. Also, coconut oil promotes the loss of belly fat and aids in weight loss.

Cottage Cheese and Greek Yogurt

Cottage cheese and Greek yogurt are extremely high in protein. While these items may have some small amounts carbohydrates, they still are included in this diet. For 5 ounces of Greek yogurt offers 5 grams of carbohydrates and 11 grams of protein. The same amount of cottage cheese provides 18 grams of protein, along with 5 grams of carbs.

Both products have shown that they help decrease your appetite and promote a feeling of being full. Cottage cheese and Greek yogurt can be joined with crushed nuts, sugar-free sweetener, or cinnamon.

Olive Oil offers fantastic benefits for your heart. It is extremely high in oleic acid, as well as monounsaturated fat. This product also provides a lower risk of developing heart disease. In addition, olive oil also offers a high level of antioxidants that are known as phenols. This compound will help further to protect the heart by decreasing any inflammation, as well as improve the artery functions. Olive oil is a pure source of fat, which means it includes no carbs. It is the perfect base for a home-made salad dressing.

Seeds and Nuts

Seeds and nuts are incredibly healthy. They are exceptionally low in carbohydrates and high in fat. Frequently eating nuts has been shown to reduce the risk factors of heart disease, depression, cancer, and other chronic type diseases.

Since seeds and nuts are extremely high in fiber, you will feel fuller, longer. You will absorb fewer calories overall. Even though seeds and nuts are exceptionally low in net carbs, the amount will vary drastically depending on the type of seed or nut. For one ounce of a popular nut, it will contain about 28 carbohydrates.

- Almonds: 6 grams of carbs — 3 grams net

- Brazil: 3 grams of carbs — 1 gram's net

- Cashews: 9 grams of carbs — 8 grams net

- Macadamia: 4 grams of carbs — 2 grams net

- Pecans: 4 grams of carbs — 1 gram's net

- Pistachios: 8 grams of carbs — 5 grams net

- Walnuts: 4 grams of carbs — 2 grams net

- Chia Seeds: 12 grams of carbs — 1 gram's net

- Flaxseeds: 8 grams of carbs — 0 grams net

- Pumpkin Seeds: 5 grams of carbs — 4 grams net

- Sesame Seeds: 7 grams of carbs — 3 grams net

Berries

Most of the fruits that are typically eaten are way too high in carbohydrates. Therefore, they are not able to be included in this diet. Berries are the exception. They are exceptionally low in carbohydrates and extremely high in fiber. Blackberries and raspberries have just as much fiber as they do other nutrients.

These two fruits contain many antioxidants and have been known to reduce inflammation and protects against diseases. In a serving size of 3.5 ounces, this list shows you the net content of carbohydrates.

- Blackberries: 10 grams of carbs — 5 grams net

- Blueberries 12 grams of carbs — 12 grams net

- Raspberries: 12 grams of carbs — 6 grams net

- Strawberries: 8 grams of carbs — 6 grams net

Cream and Butter

Cream and butter are great fats to include in your diet. Each of them contains only a few carbs in each serving. For years, cream and butter were believed to contribute or cause heart disease due to their saturated fat content. However, many studies later, it has been proven that many people saturated fat is not linked to heart disease.

Some studies have been conducted that show moderate consumption of dairy may reduce the risk of stroke and heart attacks. Like many other dairy products that are high in fat, cream and butter are extraordinarily rich in linoleum acid, which promotes fat loss in the body.

Shirataki Noodles

These types of noodles are a great food to eat on the Keto diet. Shirataki noodles are made from viscous fibers called glucomannan. They absorb up to fifty times more weight in water. The viscous fiber will form a gel that will slow down the movement of the food through the digestive tract. This will help decrease the feeling of hunger and reduces sugar spikes. It is a beneficial way to lose weight and manage diabetes. Forms of shirataki noodles include rice, linguine, and fettuccine. They can be substituted for other types of noodles in recipes.

Olives

Olives offer the same type of health benefits as olive oil. However, these are in solid form. The main antioxidant in these tasty little Morales is called European. It offers anti-inflammatory properties and can protect the body cells from any damage. In addition, there are studies that show

45

that eating olives will help prevent high blood pressure and bone loss. For one ounce of olives, you will eat 2 grams of carbohydrates, as well as fiber.

Unsweetened Tea and Coffee

Tea and coffee are great healthy drinks that contain no carbs. They do contain caffeine, which increases the body's metabolism and can improve physical performance, mood, and alertness. They have also been shown to reduce diabetes. In fact, it has been proven that people that consume high levels of caffeine have a lower risk of developing diabetes.

Adding in some heavy cream to tea or coffee is acceptable, but you will need to stay away from products that use the word "light." Typically, it is the products that are advertised as non-fat. They contain a lot of carbohydrates.

Cocoa Powder and Dark Chocolate

Cocoa and dark chocolate are delicious and offer a high number of antioxidants. Cocoa is considered a super fruit. Dark chocolate has many flavanols, which reduce heart disease risks. It lowers the blood pressure and will keep your arteries healthy.

Surprisingly, chocolate can be included in the Keto diet. However, it is crucial that you eat dark chocolate. It should contain a minimum amount of 70 percent of cocoa solids. One ounce of unsweetened chocolate includes 3 grams of carbohydrates. That means no milk, chocolate candy bars!

Foods to Avoid

All types of sweetened beverages, fruit juices, and other sweetened drinks.

All types of starchy vegetables including white potatoes, sweet potatoes, etc.

Commercial fried foods, snacks, and bakery products including sugar-based desserts.

Wheat pasta, bread, rice, cereals, and other high carb wheat products.

All types of commercial processed food items.

Legumes and beans

Fruits can be consumed but a small quantity

Alcohol and unhealthy cooking oils

Here are some things that should always be on your list:

Butter

Butter is quite healthy! The good news is that you can get a ton of fat-soluble vitamins with butter and this is an especially important part of your Keto Diet. Make sure that you are getting lots of great organic butter. Some of the top brands include Organic Valley, Vital Farms, and Kerry gold. The dairy free alternative to butter is ghee, and this is essentially clarified butter with the milk solids removed. The deeper the color of the butter, the better that it is for you.

Coconut Oil

We have talked about coconut oil before and why it is great for cooking along with all the other different benefits of this food. The good news is that you can get it wherever you are shopping these days. The goal is making sure that you are getting virgin, cold-pressed, and/or unrefined coconut oil. Nature's Way is one of the leading brands with coconut oil, so if you are looking for something that is a known quantity, this is a great one to use.

Lard or Tallow

Animal fats are always better for you than plant fats and they form the foundation of your Keto Diet. Lard is rendered pig fat and tallow is fat that is rendered from animals like cows, sheep, and lambs. This low polyunsaturated fat is the better fat to cook with and that means you get the most out of your meal prep. Quality is always the greater concern than quantity, so you want to be sure that you are taking the time needed to find some great sources. One of the best sources is Epic Beef Tallow.

Avocados

When it comes to a Keto food that does it all, there are few that can measure up to the avocado. The avocado takes literally no time to prepare and is probably the easiest side dish ever. Some will say that the avocado has a ton of carbs, but the avocado is also fiber rich, which means that in terms of net carbs, the medium avocado only has about three grams of these net carbs. When starting the Keto Diet, the avocado is a great tool for the transition and will help you counter the Keto flu.

Nuts

When it comes to snacking, there are very few nuts that do not do the job. Nuts in moderation are very keto friendly and they are associated with lower rates to type 2 diabetes. Make sure that the nuts are raw so that you are not getting carbs in an unintended way.

Heavy Cream

For people who love coffee, getting rid of half and half is tough, however heavy cream is a more than suitable alternative. Creamers are positively awful for the Keto Diet, so make sure to use heavy cream along with some flavored stevia to up the ante.

Cheese

How many diets are there telling you to eat cheese? The reality is that any cheese that is made from raw milk is the key to having a great cheese. The good news is that most grocery stores have these cheeses. The goal is making sure that you see the words "unpasteurized" and "raw" on the list of the different ingredients that are used to make the cheese.

Beef

In terms of a source of protein, there are few that do a better job than beef. It has a higher content of fat than fish, chicken, and most of the different cuts of pork, so you will hit your macros much easier. Also, when you are looking for iron, there are few things that are better than beef – it has tons of naturally occurring iron.

Chicken

What is crazy is that chicken has become one of the biggest foods in America. Over nearly 60 years, chicken consumption has risen by nearly 400% which means that everyone loves this poultry. The great thing about the Keto Diet is that you want the fatty cuts of chicken, and that means chicken thighs – the most flavorful part of the bird.

Pork

Pork is vital and bacon is a big part of it, and with the massive amount of Vitamin B that is found in pork, you will certainly enjoy eating this food and getting all the nutrients that are found within it.

Fatty Fish

Fish is one of the best ways to get your omega-3 fatty acids and most Americans are not doing enough when it comes to getting this nutrient. The best fish for this are sardines, herring, mackerel, and salmon. Get at least one serving of fish per week but if you can do up to 2 to 3 servings, you will be well served on your Keto Diet. Fish has so many different things going for it, and you should make it a big part of your experience with the Keto Diet.

Eggs

When it comes to a food that is good on a budget and has a ton of nutrients, there are few things that can do the job like the incredible edible egg. One thing that eggs have a lot of is choline. Americans are terrible at getting choline and when you have four eggs each day, you get the right amount of choline for your daily needs. That being said, an easy way to get eggs in a cheap way is get the eggs that are from your local farmers. The farmer's market gives you fresher eggs that have more nutritional value than the eggs found under the lights in the supermarket. Plus, many of these eggs are pasture raised, which means that they have the most nutritional value available.

Almond Butter

Almost butter and other nut butters are an awesome treat and if you look at the ingredients, you have a winner if the ingredients that you are seeing are simply nuts and salt. These are the best types of nut butters. The ubiquitous brands of nut butters such as peanut butter all have sugar added, and that means you are having to deal with the different issues that come with increasing your blood sugar, which is what you do not want on the Keto Diet.

Blackberries

The reality is that fruit is difficult to have with the Keto Diet because the amount of carbs that you are taking in will add up so what you need to do is get low-sugar fruit and the best fruits for this are berries. Blackberries are fantastic for this reason; they have a ton of antioxidants and can add a ton of flavor to the Keto Diet. If you are looking for a snack, there are few things that can do the job better than some blackberries and cream. The best time to buy blackberries are when they are in season, they have robust flavor and are excellent in terms of aromatic qualities as well.

Raspberries

Just like blackberries have loads of great qualities, raspberries are also great as well. They have an absurdly low 7 grams of carbs per cup and like all berries, they have tons of antioxidants and flavonoids. The reason why you should have them in your diet, besides their properties? Raspberries are a great and often underrated flavor.

Broccoli

When it comes to vegetables that soak up the cooking fat, there are few vegetables that do the job quite like broccoli. Butter gives broccoli some excellent flavor and allows you to hit your fat macros for the day. Also, when it comes to vitamins and minerals, there are few vegetables that pack as much of a punch as broccoli.

Spinach

One of the best leafy green vegetables to get is spinach. Along with kale, collard greens, and cabbage, these dark leafy greens are dens with nutrients and have a ton of minerals. When it comes to salads and omelets though, spinach does a much better job than the other dark leafy greens. Again, one of the best things to do is get the spinach and other dark leafy greens from the local farmer's market. These locally sourced ingredients will do a great job in getting you the nutrients that you need.

Asparagus

Asparagus is one of the best foods because it has only two grams of net carbs per cup, this is insane. It also pairs great with steak as well. When it comes to a vegetable that not only looks the part but performs its function with admirable levels of efficiency, asparagus has few peers.

Brussels Sprouts

The problem with Brussel sprouts is that the carbs will quickly add up with them, so you must be smart. In a single cup, there are about 8 grams of carbs in them, so make sure that when you are adding Brussel sprouts to your meal that you take this into consideration so that you don't throw off your macros that you have worked so hard on.

Cauliflower

There are a lot of people who find cauliflower to be one of the most versatile foods out there. It is turned into pizza crusts and makes healthy versions of the different foods that we enjoy. So, if you are looking for something that can essentially replace some of the bad parts of your favorite foods, this is a great substitute. Cauliflower does a great job in substituting the way that grains work so you can replicate the stuff that you love.

Dark Chocolate

When it comes to a food that may not seem like it should be part of the Keto Diet but has tons of great stuff, that is what dark chocolate is. The good thing is that you can get chocolate that has higher percentages of cocoa. The most palatable dark chocolate is 85% cocoa to 95% cocoa. There are also chocolates that are sweetened with the Keto Diet friendly sweeteners. One of the brands that is most well-known for getting this done is Lily's. They do an excellent job with chocolate for the Keto Diet.

Chapter 8: Meal Recipes (with images)

Breakfast Recipes

Green banana pancakes

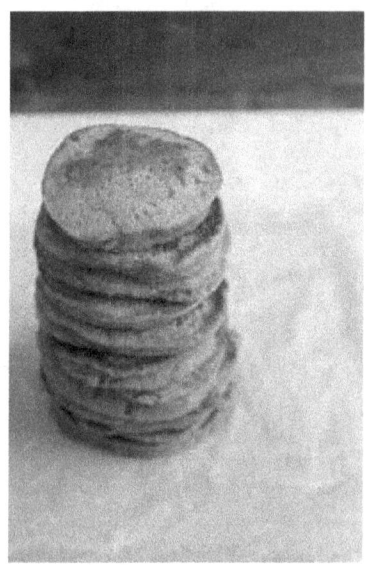

Total time: 20 minutes

Ingredients:

- ☐ 2 large peeled bananas
- ☐ 2 eggs
- ☐ 6 tablespoons of coconut flour
- ☐ 2 teaspoons cassava flour or arrowroot starch
- ☐ Pinch of salt
- ☐ ¼ teaspoon stevia powder
- ☐ 1 tablespoon of baking powder
- ☐ Coconut oil or grass-fed butter

Directions

Mash the banana till its smooth

In another bowl, mix the coconut flour, stevia, arrowroot, or cassava, baking soda, and pinch of salt to make a powder mix

Crack and whisk your egg very lightly.

Pour into the banana and mix up

Pour in the powder mix to the banana and egg [If the mix is too thick, pour in little water at a time. Use a spoon to pour in water.]

Preheat a skillet. Rub the warm skillet with your butter, ghee, or oil.

Pour in your batter to the skillet with a spoon

When it is golden brown on the outside, flip it and let it cool

Serve warm

Berry bread spread

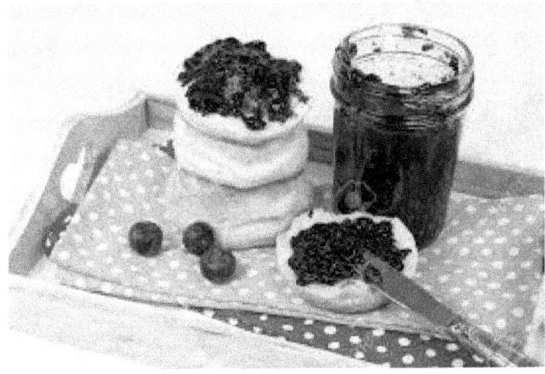

Total time: 15 minutes

Ingredients:

- ☐ 2 cups of coconut cream
- ☐ 2 ounces of strawberries
- ☐ 1 ½ ounces of blueberries

- ☐ 1 ½ ounces of raspberries
- ☐ ½ teaspoon coconut extract

Directions

Separate 3 of each berry type and dice in small pieces

Put in the strawberries, blueberries, and raspberries in a blender till its smooth

Pour out and mix with coconut extract and coconut cream

Mix till smooth and blend again

Pour in diced berries

Serve

Chocolate bread spread

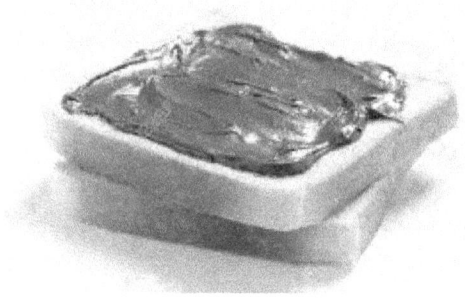

Total time: 20 minutes

Ingredients:

- ☐ 4 cups of sweet cream
- ☐ 2 ounces of coconut oil
- ☐ 3 ounces of chocolate
- ☐ 1 teaspoon of coconut extract

- ☐ 1 tablespoon of powdered cacao
- ☐ Groundnuts [optional]

Directions

Place sweet cream in a microwavable bowl and heat for 10-15 seconds

Pour in coconut oil and stir

Put in chocolate and cacao

Put in microwave for a little under a minute

When it is warm, you can put in your groundnuts if you want them in

Place in bowls and refrigerate

Keto almond cereal

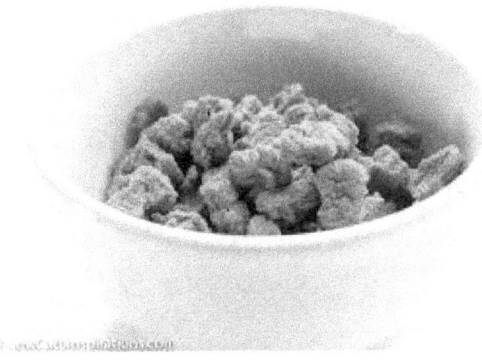

Total time: 25 minutes

Ingredients:

- ☐ 3 cups of unsweetened coconut flakes
- ☐ 1 cup of sliced almonds
- ☐ ¾ tablespoon of cinnamon
- ☐ ¾ tablespoon of nutmeg

Directions

Preheat oven to 250 degrees F

The almonds and coconut flakes together

Pour in the nutmeg and cinnamon

Put on a baking tray at bake for 3-5 minutes

Depending on the thickness of your coconut, it can be ready sooner. Take off when slightly brown

Enjoy with milk

Keto granola cereal

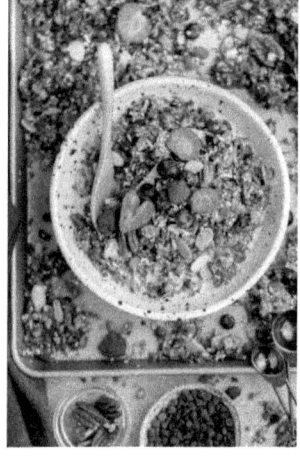

Total time: 35 minutes

Ingredients:

☐   1 cup of flaxseeds

Directions

Beat the egg

Preheat oven to 300 degrees F

Set out a bowl and put in all ingredients

Set out a baking pan with parchment paper

Pour ingredients in

Bake for 30 minutes

Keto fruit cereal

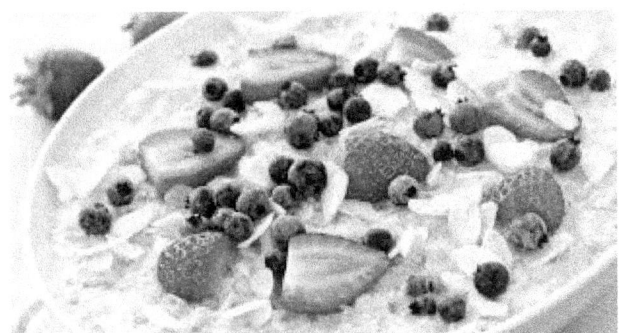

Total time: 25 minutes

Ingredients:

- ☐   1 cup of coconut flakes

- ☐   ½ cup of sliced strawberries

- ☐   ¼ cup of sliced raspberries

- ☐

Directions

Preheat oven to 300 degrees F

Set out a baking pan with parchment paper

Pour the flakes in

Bake for 5 minutes

Pour in sliced raspberries and strawberries.

Enjoy with almond milk

Keto chicken and avocado

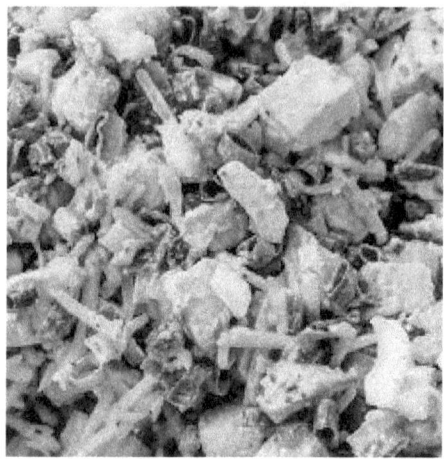

Total time: 25 minutes

Ingredients:

☐   6 medium-sized pieces of chicken. Boneless.

☐   1 avocado

☐   2 eggs

☐   Keto Mayo

☐   Salt

☐   Pepper

☐   Ground Garlic

☐   1/8 cup of olive oil

Directions

Soft boil 2 eggs

Put the seasonings together in a bowl

Sprinkle them generously on the chicken.

Cover for 5 minutes

Heat up the olive oil and fry the chicken

Take out the chicken and set aside

Cut avocado in two and remove the pit

Dice on half and set aside

Slice the eggs in half so you have four pieces

Sprinkle a little salt on the avocados [optional]

Spread mayo on the chicken [optional]

On a place, set your eggs, meat, and avocados. Enjoy warm

Keto almond pancake

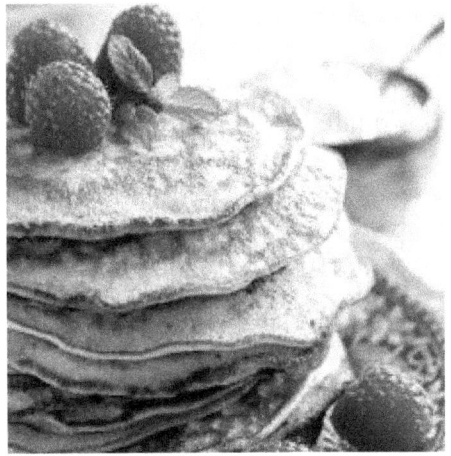

Total time: 30 minutes

Ingredients:

- 1 ½ cups of almond flour
- 3 teaspoons of baking powder

- 1 teaspoon of salt
- 1 tablespoon of stevia
- 1 ¼ cup of almond milk
- 1 egg
- 3 tablespoons of melted ghee
- 2 teaspoons of olive oil

Directions

Put in dry ingredients and stir.

In another bowl, mix egg and mix

Pour the wet inside the dry and add the butter.

Mix well

Heat a frying pan and

Pour in olive oil to the pot at teaspoon at a time

Pour in the batter and brown each side equally

Serve warm

Keto meat balls

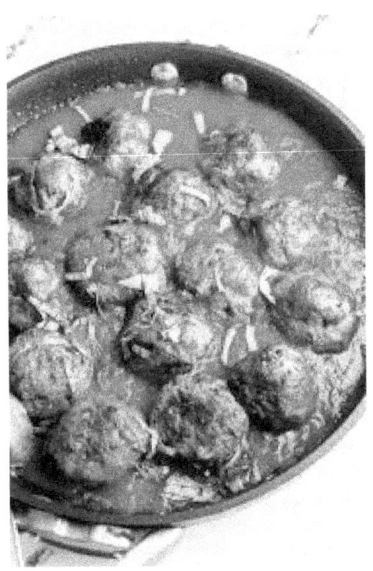

Total time: 35 minutes

Ingredients:

- ☐ 11 eggs
- ☐ 7 ounces of mozzarella cheese
- ☐ 4 ounces of chopped and cooked bacon
- ☐ 3 chopped scallions
- ☐ 1 ounce of ground beef
- ☐ Salt
- ☐ **Pepper**
- ☐ Teaspoon of olive oil

Directions

Preheat oven to 350 degrees F

Spray baking spray on your muffin tin

Put the scallions evenly in the tin. Let them be at the bottom

In a bowl, mix eggs and add a teaspoon of oil

Pour in cheese and add salt and pepper to taste.

In another bowl, mix bacon and chicken

Pour it into cheese and stir

Pour the mix into the tray and bake for 17-20 minutes

Keto scrambled eggs

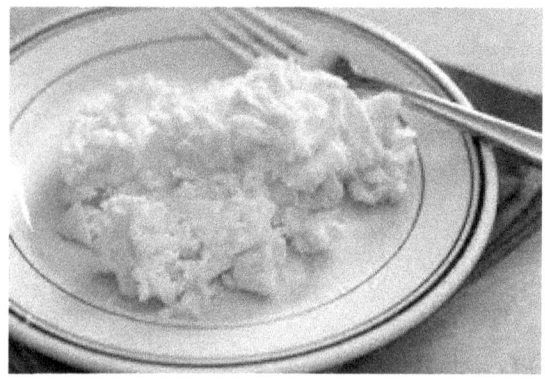

Total time: 15 minutes

Ingredients:

- 3 eggs
- 1 ounce of ghee
- Salt and pepper

Directions

Crack eggs and mix with salt and pepper

Heat skillet and pour in butter'

When slightly melted, pour in eggs and scramble

Banana Waffles

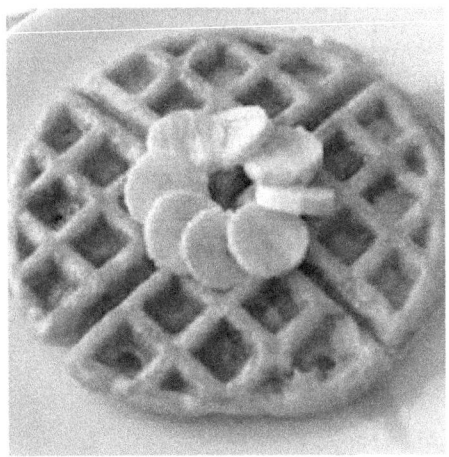

Total time: 35 minutes

Ingredients:

4 eggs

1 ripe banana

¾ cup coconut milk

¾ cup almond flour

1 pinch of salt

1 tbsp. of ground psyllium husk powder

½ tsp. vanilla extract

1 tsp. baking powder

1 tsp. of ground cinnamon

Butter or coconut oil for frying

Directions:

Mash the banana thoroughly until you get a mashed potato consistency.

Add all the other ingredients in and whisk thoroughly to evenly distribute the dry and wet ingredients. You should be able to get a pancake-like consistency

Fry the waffles in a pan or use a waffle maker.

You can serve it with hazelnut spread and fresh berries. Enjoy!

Keto Cinnamon Coffee

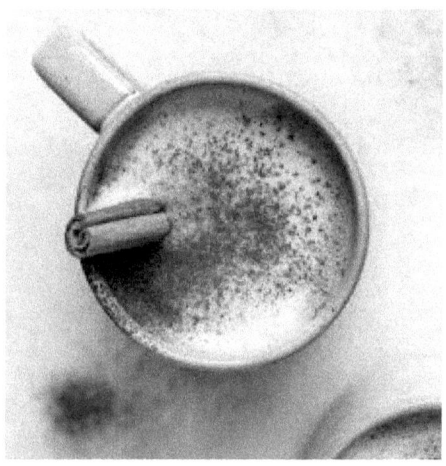

Total time: 10 minutes

Ingredients:

2 tbsp. ground coffee

1/3 cup heavy whipping cream

1 tsp. ground cinnamon

2 cups water

Directions:

Start by mixing the cinnamon with the ground coffee.

Pour in hot water and do what you usually do when brewing.

Use a mixer or whisk to whip the cream 'til you get stiff peaks

Serve in a tall mug and put the whipped cream on the surface. Sprinkle with some cinnamon and enjoy.

Keto Waffles and Blueberries

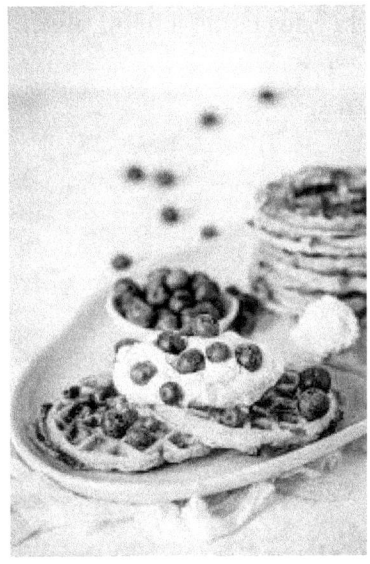

Total time: 20 minutes

Ingredients:

8 eggs

5 oz. melted butter

1 tsp. vanilla extract

2 tsp. baking powder

1/3 cup coconut flour

3 oz. butter (topping)

1 oz. fresh blueberries (topping)

Directions:

Start by mixing the butter and eggs first until you get a smooth batter. Put in the remaining ingredients except those that we will be using as topping.

Heat your waffle iron to medium temperature and start pouring in the batter for cooking

In a separate bowl, mix the butter and blueberries using a hand mixer. Use this to top off your freshly cooked waffles

Baked Avocado Eggs

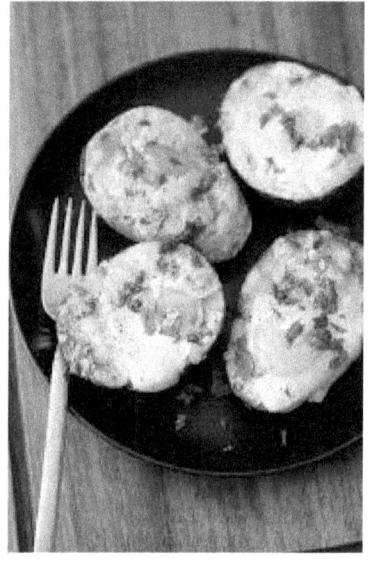

Total time: 35 minutes

Ingredients:

2 avocados

4 eggs

½ cup bacon bits, around 55 grams

2 tbsp. fresh chives, chopped

1 sprig of chopped fresh basil, chopped

1 cherry tomato, quartered

Salt and pepper to taste

Shredded cheddar cheese

Directions:

Start by preheating the oven to 400 degrees Fahrenheit

Slice the avocado and remove the pits. Put them on a baking sheet and crack some eggs onto the center hole of the avocado. If it is too small, just scoop out more of the flesh to make room. Salt and pepper to taste.

Top with bacon bits and bake for 15 minutes.

Remove and sprinkle with herbs. Enjoy!

Mushroom Omelet

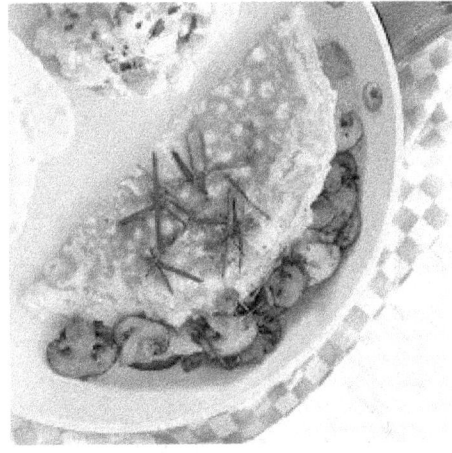

Total time: 10 minutes

Ingredients:

3 eggs, medium

1 oz. shredded cheese

1 oz. butter used for frying

¼ yellow onion, chopped

4 large sliced mushrooms

Your favorite vegetables, optional

Salt and pepper to taste

Directions:

Crack and whisk the eggs in a bowl. Add some salt and pepper to taste.

Melt the butter in a pan using low heat. Put in the mushroom and onion, cooking the two until you get that amazing smell.

Pour the egg mix into the pan and allow it to cook on medium heat.

Allow the bottom part to cook before sprinkling the cheese on top of the still-raw portion of the egg.

Carefully pry the edges of the omelet and fold it in half. Allow it to cook for a few more seconds before removing the pan from the heat and sliding it directly onto your plate.

Soft Boiled Keto Eggs

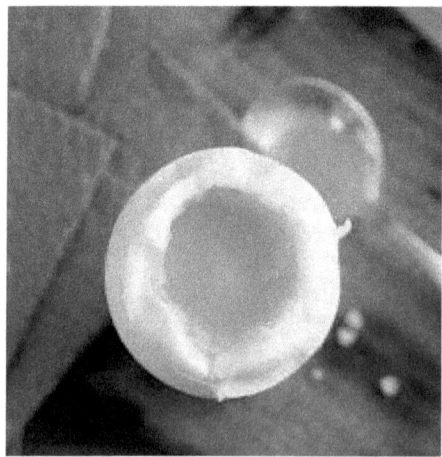

Total time: 20 minutes

Ingredients:

3 large eggs

1 tbsp. of unsalted butter

¼ tsp. thyme leaves

Freshly ground black pepper

Salt to taste

Directions:

Grab a saucepan and fill it halfway with water, apply high heat until the water boils.

When boiling, gently place the eggs in the water. Set a timer for 6 minutes.

Take on tablespoon of butter and put it in the microwave for around 20 seconds or until it melts.

Remove the eggs from the saucepan, carefully pouring the hot water in the sink. This is great because the hot water can also help remove clogs from your pipes!

Carefully take a bowl and fill it with cold water. Put the eggs inside so it can cool off. Once done, peel the egg and place it in your bowl of melted butter.

Add salt and pepper to taste and thyme for garnishing. Make sure to eat it while fresh!

French Omelet

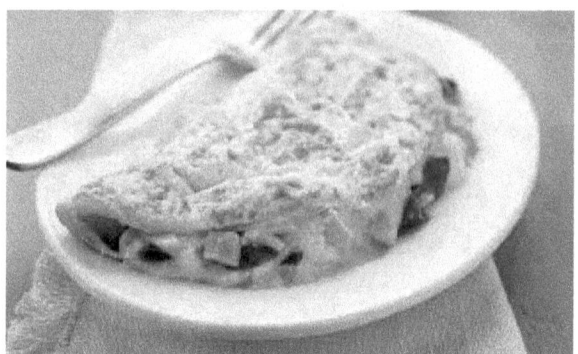

Total time: 30 minutes

Ingredients:

2 large eggs

4 large egg whites

¼ cup fat-free milk

¼ cup cubed ham, cooked

¼ cup cheddar cheese, shredded

1/8 tsp. salt

1/8 tsp. pepper

1 tbsp. onion, chopped

1 tbsp. green pepper, chopped

Directions:

Whisk together the eggs and egg whites until blended.

Add the salt, pepper, and milk, mixing them together until fully blended.

Using medium heat, coat your skillet with cooking spray and pour the egg mixture in when the surface is hot and ready.

As it cooks, push it around the edges so the uncooked portion flows around until there are no runny liquid on top.

When it is already around ¾ cooked, put all the remaining ingredients on top and continue cooking until done.

Apple Chicken Sausage

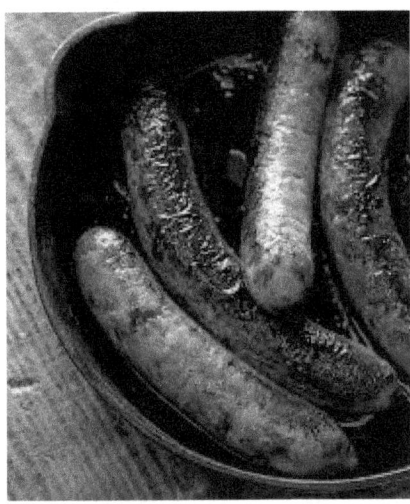

Total time: 35 minutes

Ingredients:

1 large tart apple, diced

1-pound ground chicken

¼ tsp. pepper

1 tsp. salt

2 tsp. poultry seasoning

Directions:

Grab a large bowl and combine all the ingredients except the ground chicken

Combine the chicken in the mix and blend well. Create a total of 8 patties of similar sizes which should be around 3 inches in diameter each.

Cook them up using medium heat. Make sure each side gets around 5 to 6 minutes of cooking time.

Keto Cereal

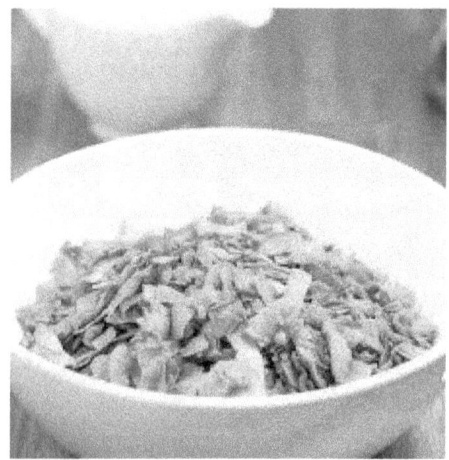

Total time: 1 hours 20 minutes

Ingredients:

1 cup shredded coconut, unsweetened

1 cup flaked coconut, unsweetened

½ cup flaxseeds

½ cup flaked almonds

1/3 cup Pepitas

1/3 cup sunflower seeds

1/3 cup chia seeds

1/3 cup erythritol

1/3 cup melted coconut oil

1 tbsp. ground cinnamon

1 tsp. vanilla extract

Directions:

Preheat your over to 150 degrees Celsius or 300 degrees Fahrenheit

Mix all the ingredients together in one convenient bowl.

Once they are combined, spread them over a pan on top of a lined cookie sheet

Bake them for 25 to 35 minutes. You might have to take them out every five minutes and stir up the mix to prevent burning.

The goal is to create an even golden brown or have them reach that lightly toasted color. Once you have got that, remove them from the oven.

Allow to cool and break them up and store in an airtight container.

Keto Breakfast Burrito

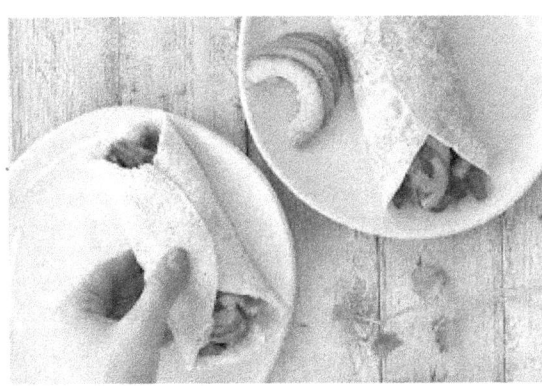

Total time: 20 minutes

Ingredients:

1 tbsp butter

2 eggs medium

2 tbsp full fat cream

choice of herbs or spices

salt and pepper to taste

Directions:

Grab a bowl and whisk the eggs and cream together. Add your choice of herbs and spices, depending on personal preferences.

Melt the butter in a frying pan using low to medium heat.

Pour the egg mixture into the pan.

Cook and swirl to create a thin layer of egg burrito.

Gently lift the egg burrito from the frying pan. Put the fillings you want inside and roll it up. Enjoy!

Lunch Recipes

Baked lamb ribs macadamia with tomato salsa

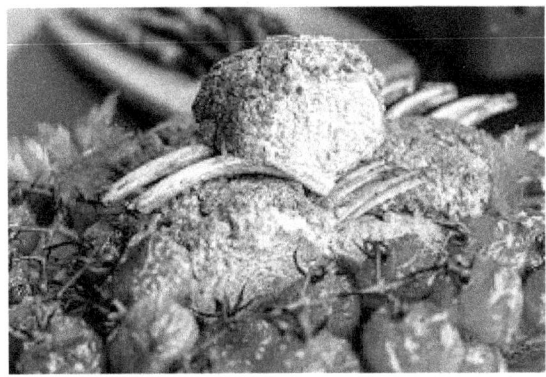

Total time: 45 minutes

Ingredients:

- ½ pound of fresh lamb ribs

- ½ cup of cherry tomatoes

- ½ teaspoon pepper

- ½ cup of macadamia

- ½ tablespoon of macadamia oil

- ¼ cup fresh parsley

- 1 teaspoon of balsamic vinegar

- 1 teaspoon of minced garlic

- 2 tablespoons of extra virgin olive oil

Directions

Cut up the lamb ribs into stripes or pieces

Preheat your oven to 204°C. Ensure that your baking tray is lined with aluminum foil.

Place the macadamia, garlic, parsley, pepper, and olive oil, in the food processor. Blend till the mixture is smooth and lump free.

Rub your processed mixture all over your cut lamb pieces. Ensure that it is coated well enough.

Arrange your strips nicely in the baking tray and bake for 20-25 minutes.

While the lamb bakes, cut the cherry in pieces. You can cut each into four then place them in an aluminum cup.

Pour macadamia oil on the tomatoes. Use spoon to mix the oil and tomatoes without squishing it. The aim is to get the oil all over it.

Take out your lamp and place on a plate.

Place your tomatoes in the oven for 4-5 minutes.

Take out the tomatoes and pour sparse amounts of balsamic vinegar and stir.

Pour the tomatoes on the lamb and serve warm.

Grilled Garlic Butter Shrimp

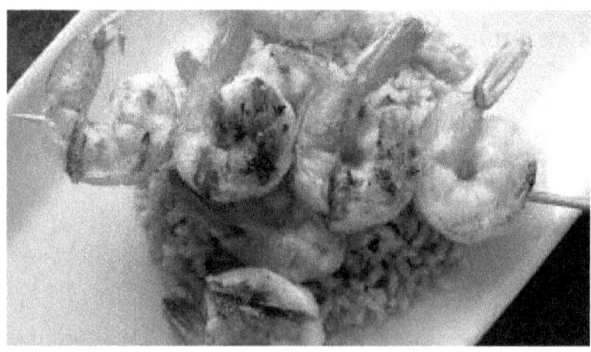

Total time: 35 minutes

Ingredients:

- ☐ 1 pound of large shrimps
- ☐ 1¼ tablespoon of minced garlic
- ☐ 1 teaspoon minced parsley, minced
- ☐ ½ cup of butter
- ☐ Salt and pepper
- ☐ Bamboo skewers

Directions

Defreeze, peel, and devein the shrimp. Be careful not to take off the tails.

Preheat the grill to medium heat. This should be around 360°F

Melt your butter.

Mix the melted butter with garlic. Add salt and pepper to your taste.

Put your bamboo skewers through the shrimp

Once grill is heated, place the shrimp on it and start cooking. Turn the shrimp over after 2 minutes.

Spread your garlic and butter mixture on the side facing you.

After two minutes, turn it over and spread the garlic and butter mix on the other side

After you have flipped the shrimp, baste the side facing up with the garlic butter sauce.

Ensure both sides are evenly cooked.

Remove the shrimp and serve

Tomato Chili Chicken Tender with Fresh Basils

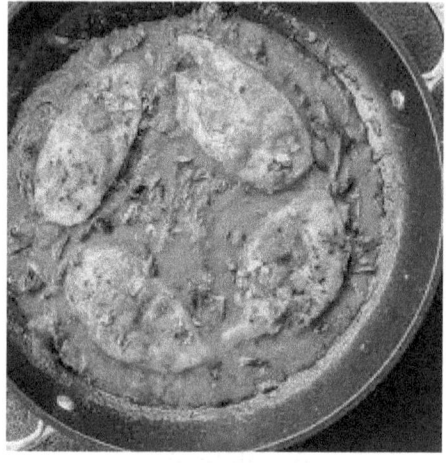

Total time: 50 minutes

Ingredients:

- 2 pounds of boneless chicken thighs
- 4 tablespoons extra virgin olive oil
- 3 lemon grasses
- 3 tablespoons red chili flakes
- 2½ tablespoons minced garlic
- 2 cups water
- ¼ cup sliced red tomatoes
- ½ cup fresh basils
- Salt and pepper

Directions

Defreeze your chicken

Cut the chicken into small to medium pieces

Place the pieces in a skillet

Add some minced garlic and lemon grass

Add some salt and pepper to taste

Pour water over the chicken

Boil the chicken till the water totally/almost totally evaporates

Take out the chicken and set it aside

Heat a saucepan and pour olive oil in

Place the chicken and let it cook till it is brown

Place your tomatoes, basils, and chili flakes

Serve warm

Pork crack slaw

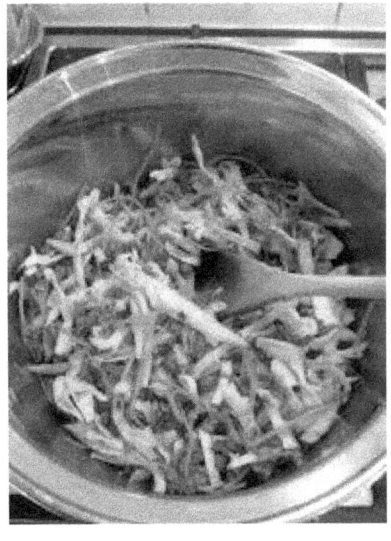

Total time: 30 minutes

Ingredients:

☐   1 pound of ground pork sausage

- [ ] 1 teaspoon of mixed garlic

- [ ] 1 Bags of ready-mix dry coleslaw

- [ ] 1 teaspoon of sesame oil

- [ ] 2 tablespoons of rice vinegar

- [ ] ¼ of a red onion

- [ ] ¼ tablespoons of ground ginger

- [ ] Salt and pepper to taste

Directions

Place the sausage in a bowl and heat till brown and ready, place in chopped red onions while you heat

When the sausage is ready, pour in the rice vinegar, sesame oil, minced garlic, coleslaw kits and salt and pepper to taste.

Stir on fore for five to seven minutes to enable everything cook

Pour in the soy sauce and cover the pot.

Let the contents steam for 5 to ten minutes

While it steams, dice half or a green onion and slice the other half to serve

Take it out and serve warm

Keto lasagna

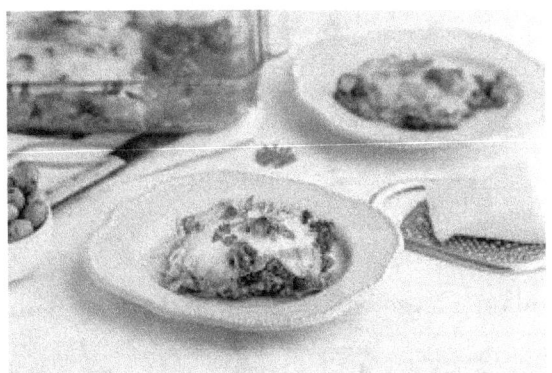

Total time: 30 minutes

Ingredients:

- [ ] 16 ounces of ricotta
- [ ] 8 ounces block cream cheese
- [ ] 4 cups of shredded mozzarella
- [ ] 4 minced cloves of garlic
- [ ] 3 large eggs
- [ ] 2 cups of freshly grated Parmesan cheese
- [ ] 1 tablespoon of extra virgin olive oil
- [ ] 1 ½ tablespoons of tomato paste
- [ ] 1 ½ ground beef
- [ ] ¾ cups of marinara
- [ ] ½ white or yellow onion
- [ ] 1 tablespoon of dried oregano
- [ ] Cooking spray, butter, or oil

- [ ] Pinch crushed red pepper flakes

- [ ] Chopped parsley

- [ ] Black pepper

- [ ] Kosher salt

Directions

Preheat the oven to about 350° F

Lay a cooing parchment or foil on a large baking sheet and grease with cooking oil, or butter.

In another bowl, put in 2 ½ cups of mozzarella, 8 ounces of cheese, and 1 cup of parmesan cheese. Put in all the eggs and mix very well. Add salt and pepper to taste.

Pour on the baking sheet and spread it out

Bake for 15-20 minutes till its golden

Heat some oil in large skillet

Place chopped onion and fry it until it is soft

Add the garlic after and cook for a few more minutes

Poor in tomato paste

Heat the mixture until it is hot enough

Add salt and pepper to taste

Pour in ground beef

Cook the mixture until the meat loses its pink color

Add marinara

Put in red pepper flakes.

Cut noodles in 6 pieces.

Pour in a small amount of the sauce into a baking pan.

Then, put 2 noodles at the base. Divide the ricotta into 3. Spread one part of the ricotta over the broken noodles. Spread another part on the remaining meat and sauce which is on the top. Pour in a last part with the parmesan cheese. Make similar layers and pour cheese at the very top.

Place the mix in the oven until the cheese melts and the sauce heats

Sprinkle parsley and cheese if you wish

Easy meal prep chicken soup

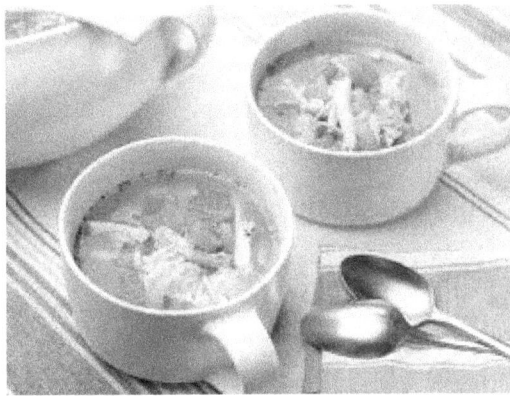

Total time: 45 minutes

Ingredients:

- 15 chicken breast tenderloins
- 2 tablespoons garlic powder
- 1 cup of chopped carrots
- 1 cup of chopped celery
- 1 tablespoon butter
- **Salt**
- Black pepper

Directions

Unfreeze chicken breast tenderloins

Place in put with 1 ½ cups of water.

Put it a teaspoon of salt

Put in ½ teaspoon of black pepper

Put in 1 tablespoon of garlic

Let the chicken boil for 20-25 minutes till soft and almost ready

Put in chopped carrots and chopped celery

Put in another tablespoon of garlic

Put in butter and cover for 5 to 10 minutes

You can freeze till needed and simply reheat when you need it.

Keto burger

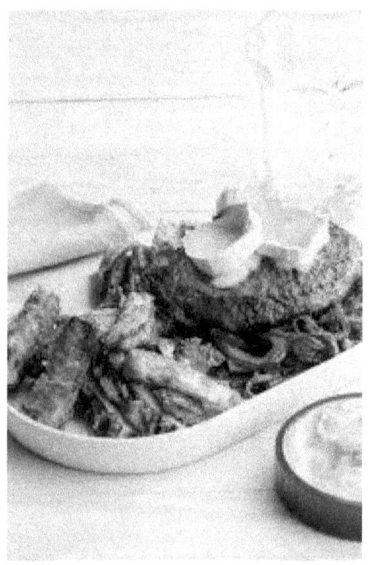

Total time: 50 minutes

Ingredients:

- ☐ 4 pounds of ground hamburger meat
- ☐ 8 tablespoons of half melted butter
- ☐ 5 cloves of garlic, minced
- ☐ 4 tablespoons Worcestershire sauce
- ☐ 1 teaspoon of ground black pepper
- ☐ 1 tablespoon of salt

Directions

Put in the meat, sauce, pepper, and garlic. Put in salt to taste.

Mix the ingredients very well with a big spoon.

Pour out the mixture on a clean board and mold into discs. Use that shape to form the mixture into patties

Put a tablespoon of butter in the center of each patty

Mold the butter into each patty

Place on a grill. Cook each side for around seven minutes

You can try cooking these burgers in foil to prevent it from catching fire due to the increased fat levels

Calamari mayo with cauliflower broccoli salad

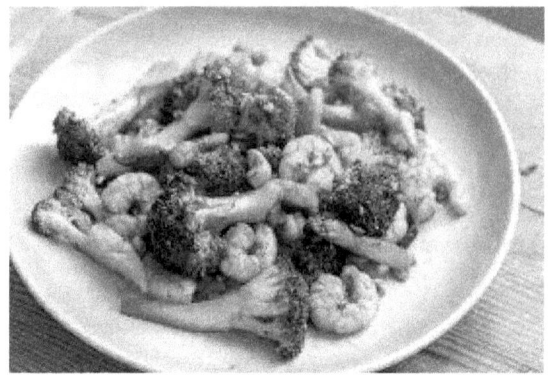

Total time: 35 minutes

Ingredients:

- 1 ½ pounds of fresh squids
- 1 ½ tablespoons of lemon juice
- 2 eggs
- 2 cups of almond flour
- 2 cups of broccoli florets
- 2 cups of cauliflower florets
- 1 cup of extra virgin olive oil
- 1 diced onion
- ½ cup diced cheddar cheese
- ½ cup of mayonnaise
- ½ teaspoon of pepper
- ½ cup of sour cream

Directions

Steam cauliflower and broccoli until they are soft and tender

Place them in bowl for later use

Remove squid ink

Crack eggs

Add salt and pepper to eggs for taste

Cut the squid into rings

Put the squid in the egg mix

Pour in almond flour

Rub in the flour into the squid and egg mix

Heat a pan and pour in oil

Fry the squid in oil until it is golden brown

Take out the squid from the oil and set it aside

In a separate bowl, put in mayonnaise, lemon juice, and sour cream

Mix well

To serve, place the fried squid on a plate with the steam broccoli and cauliflower florets then drip the mayonnaise, lemon juice, and sour cream on it

Sprinkle dry cheddar cheese

Keto strawberry rice

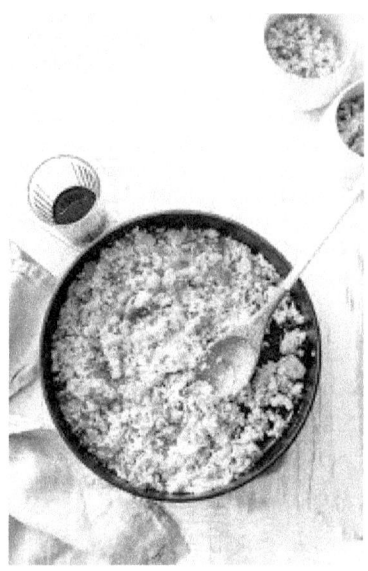

Total time: 40 minutes

Ingredients:

- ☐ 3 cups of sliced strawberries
- ☐ **Cinnamon**
- ☐ 2 cups of cooked rice
- ☐ 2 tablespoons of grass-fed butter
- ☐ 2 cup full-fat organic coconut milk
- ☐ 1 tablespoon of pure vanilla extract
- ☐ ½ cup birch xylitol
- ☐ Himalayan pink salt
- ☐ ¼ teaspoon ground

Directions

Put your 2 ½ cups of sliced strawberries, cinnamon, cooked rice, grass-fed butter, full-fat organic coconut milk, pure vanilla extract, birch xylitol, and a pinch of salt in a saucepan

Cook for 2-30 minutes while stirring till it becomes creamy

Cut up the remaining strawberries

Place the cut-up berries on the rice mixture and serve warm

Keto white rice

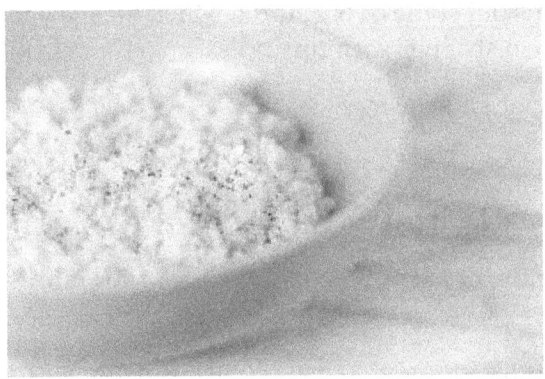

Total time: 65 minutes

Ingredients:

- [ ] 1 cup of rice
- [ ] 1 cup of diced tomatoes
- [ ] 1 ¼ cups of diced peppers
- [ ] Extra virgin olive oil ½ cup
- [ ] ½ cup of boiled ground beef
- [ ] 1/8 cup of diced green onions
- [ ] 1/8 cup of sliced spring onions
- [ ] Salt

☐   Adobo seasoning

Directions

Put 3-4 cups of water in a large saucepan and bring to boil

Put in your rice when it starts to boil and put in a tablespoon of salt

After 16-20 minutes, the rice should be ready. If you are not quite sure, you can fish it for a grain or three to taste

There should still be lots of water in the pot and so, you should strain it out. Straining the water drains out some of the starch which means you reduce the carbs. You can use a strainer with tiny holes.

Place your strained rice in a pot and cover.

Preheat your saucepan

Pour in your extra virgin oil and let it heat very slightly

Pour in your diced green onions. Fry for 15 seconds. While frying, stir it so it does not burn

Put in your spring onions and fry for another 15 seconds. Remember to stir.

Put in your pepper and stir for half a minute

Put in your tomatoes and stir.

Stir together for 5-7 minutes

Put in your boiled ground beef

Put in a teaspoon of salt

Put in a teaspoon of Adobo seasoning

Stir together for 5-8 minutes

Place your boiled rice in a serving dish.

Spread your sauce over the rice.

Enjoy hot or warm

Steamed veggies and prawn with coconut milk

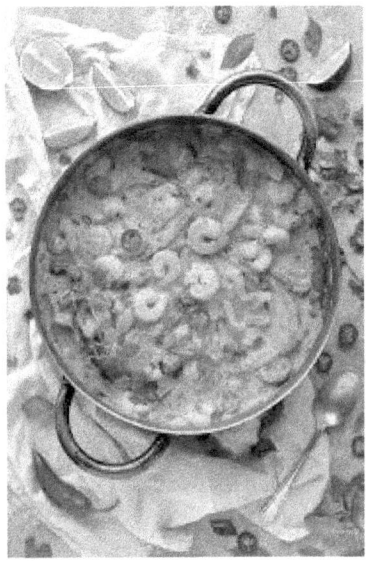

Total time: 45 minutes

Ingredients:

- ☐ 1 pound of fresh shrimps
- ☐ 4 tablespoons of extra virgin olive oil
- ☐ 1 egg
- ☐ 1/8 cup of coconut milk
- ☐ ½ cup almond flour
- ☐ ¼ cup water
- ☐ 1/8 of cup grated cheddar cheese
- ☐ 1/8 cup of diced carrot
- ☐ 1/8 of cup diced onion

□   1/8 of cup chopped leek

Directions

Peel prawns, remove heads and set aside

Crack a mix an egg in a bowl

Mix water and almond flour with water

Pour in half of the egg

Mix with a spoon

Use the mixture to make omelets

Take your peeled prawns and put them in a food processor

Process till smooth

Preheat a skillet

Pour in 1 ½ spoons of the olive oil

Put in onion and sauté. Stir fry till it is golden brown

Add the leak and carrot and stir for ten seconds

Pour in coconut milk

Stir till the milk disappears

Put the cooked veggies, prawns, and remaining half egg into the bowl

Mix well

Put an omelet on a plate and put a tablespoon of the prawn mix

Fold the omelet like an envelope

Repeat with the rest of the omelets

Preheat a saucepan and then pour the remaining olive oil into it.

When the oil is a bit hot, put the prawn envelopes in the saucepan

Cook for 2 minutes on each side till golden brown

Serve warm

Mediterranean pork chops

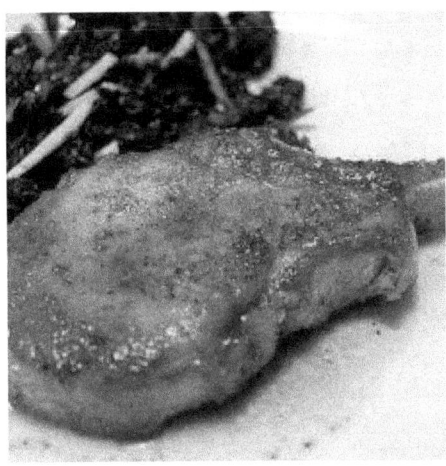

Total time: 45 minutes

Ingredients:

- ☐ 8 boneless pork loin chops
- ☐ 1 teaspoon of black pepper
- ☐ 1 teaspoon of kosher salt
- ☐ 7 minced garlic cloves
- ☐ 2 tablespoons of chopped and fresh rosemary

Directions

Mix garlic and rosemary in a bowl

Place pork chops in a bowl. Sprinkle pepper and salt

Rub in the salt and pepper

Rub in garlic and rosemary

Place pork chops in roasting pan at 425 degrees F. Do this for ten minutes

Reduce the temperature of the oven to 350 F degrees and continue roasting for about 20-25 minutes

Serve warm

Dinner Recipes

Keto Sloppy Joes

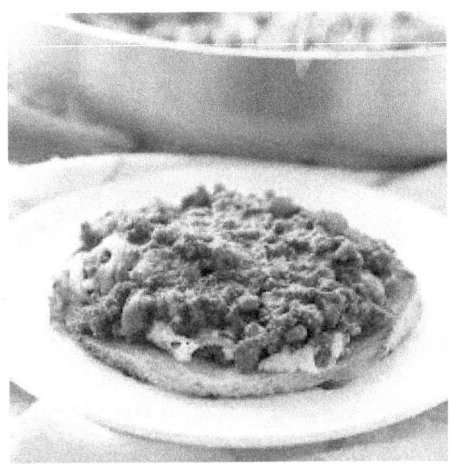

Total time: 45 minutes

Ingredients:

1 ¼ cup almond flour (for the bread)

5 tbsp. ground psyllium husk powder (for the bread)

1 tsp. sea salt (for the bread)

2 tsp. baking powder (for the bread)

2 tsp. cider vinegar (for the bread)

1 ¼ cups boiling water (for the bread)

3 egg whites (for the bread)

2 tbsp. olive oil (for the meat sauce)

1 ½ lbs. ground beef (for the meat sauce)

1 yellow onion (for the meat sauce)

4 garlic cloves (for the meat sauce)

14 oz. crushed tomatoes (for the meat sauce)

1 tbsp. chili powder (for the meat sauce)

1 tbsp. Dijon powder (for the meat sauce)

1 tbsp. red wine vinegar (for the meat sauce)

4 tbsp. tomato paste (for the meat sauce)

2 tsp. salt (for the meat sauce)

¼ tsp ground black pepper (for the meat sauce)

½ cup mayonnaise as toppings

6 oz. shredded cheese as toppings

Directions:

We are going to start by cooking the bread. First, preheat the 350 degrees Fahrenheit and then mix all the dry ingredients in a bowl.

Add some vinegar, egg whites, and boiling water in the bowl. Whisk thoroughly for 30 seconds or use a hand mixer to speed up the process. You would want a consistency that is a lot like playday

Form the dough into 5 or 8 pieces of bread. Layer then on the lowest oven rack and cook for 55 to 60 minutes.

In the meantime, you will be cooking the meat sauce. Grab a pan and cook the onion and garlic until you get that fragrant smell.

Add the ground beef and cook the meat thoroughly. Once done, add the other ingredients and cook

Allow it to simmer for 10 minutes in low heat. Add other seasonings to taste.

Low Carb Crack Slaw Egg Roll in a Bowl Recipe

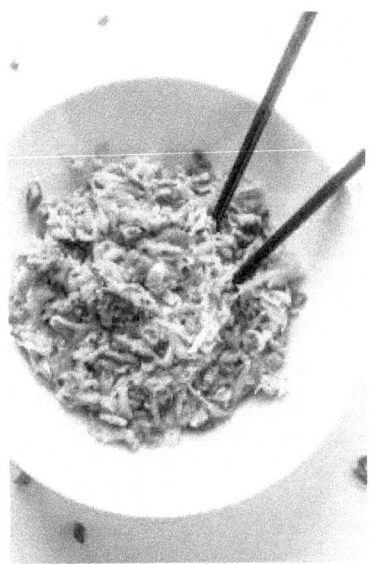

Total time: 20 minutes

Ingredients:

1 lb. ground beef

4 cups shredded coleslaw mix

1 tbsp. avocado oil

1 tsp. sea salt

¼ tsp. black pepper

4 cloves garlic, minced

3 tbsp. fresh ginger, grated

¼ cup coconut amines

2 tsp. toasted sesame oil

¼ cup green onions

Directions:

Start by heating the avocado oil in a large pan using a medium-high heat. Put in the garlic and cook for a little bit until you get that fragrant smell.

Add the ground beef and cook until it gets brownish. This should take about 10 minutes to finish. Season with salt and black pepper.

Once cooked, you can lower the heat and add the coleslaw mix and the coconut amines. Stir to cook for 5 minutes or until the coleslaw gets tender.

Remove and put in the green onions and the toasted sesame oil.

Low Carb Beef Stir Fry

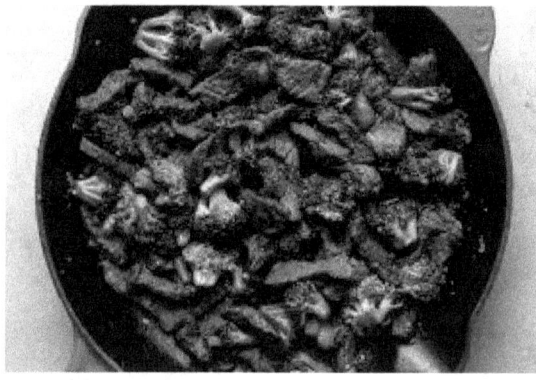

Total time: 25 minutes

Ingredients:

½ cup zucchini, spiral them into noodles about 6-inches each

¼ cup organic broccoli florets

1 bunch baby book choy, stem chopped

2 tbsp. avocado oil

2 tsp. coconut amines

1 small know of ginger, peeled, and cut

8 oz. skirt steak, thinly sliced into strips

Directions:

Heat the pan and add 1 tablespoon of oil. Sear the steak on it on high heat. This should only take around 2 minutes per side.

Reduce the heat to medium and put in the broccoli, ginger, ghee, and coconut amines. Cook for a minute, stirring as often as possible.

Add in the book choy and cook for another minute

Finally, put the zucchini into the mix and cook. Note that zucchini noodles cook quickly so you would want to pay close attention to this.

One Pan Pesto Chicken and Veggies

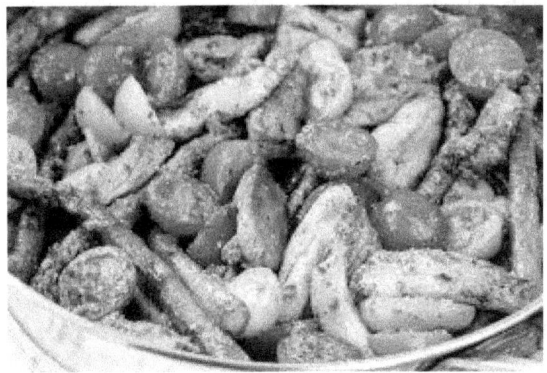

Total time: 35 minutes

Ingredients:

2 tbsp. olive oil

1 cup cherry diced tomatoes

¼ cup basil pesto

1/3 cup sun-dried tomatoes, chopped and drained

1-pound chicken thigh, bones and skinless, sliced into strips

1-pound asparagus, cut in half with the ends trimmed

Directions:

Start by heating up a large skillet. Put two tablespoons of olive oil and sliced chicken on medium heat. Season with salt and add ½ cup of the sun-dried tomatoes.

Cook for a few minutes until the chicken is cooked thoroughly. Spoon out the chicken and tomatoes and put them in a separate container.

Do not wash the skillet just yet. You will be using the oil there later.

Next, put the asparagus in the skillet and pour in the pesto. Turn the heat on medium and add the remaining sun-dried tomatoes. Cook the asparagus for 5 to 10 minutes. Put it on a separate plate when done.

Put the chicken back in the skillet and pour in pesto. Stir under medium heat for 2 minutes. You only need to reheat the chicken during this so when done, you can serve it together with the asparagus.

Crispy Peanut Tofu and Cauliflower Rice Stir-Fry

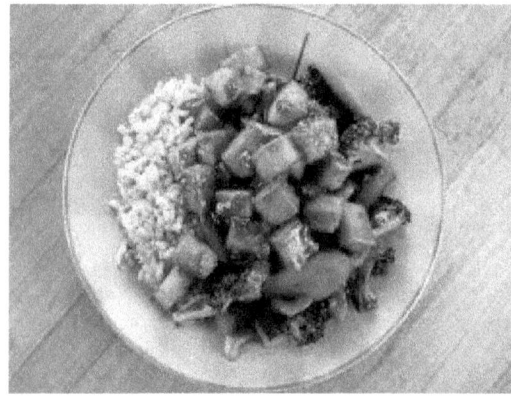

Total time: 1 hour 35 minutes

Ingredients:

12 oz. tofu, extra-firm

1 tbsp. toasted sesame oil

2 cloves minced garlic

1 small cauliflower head

1 ½ tbsp. toasted sesame oil (sauce)

½ tsp. chili garlic sauce (sauce)

2 ½ tbsp. peanut butter (sauce)

¼ cup low sodium soy sauce (sauce)

½ cup light brown sugar (sauce)

Directions:

Start by draining the tofu for 90 minutes before getting the meal ready. You can dry the tofu quickly by rolling it on an absorbent towel and putting something heavy on top. This will create a gentle pressure on the tofu to drain out the water.

Preheat the oven to 400 degrees Fahrenheit. While the oven heats up, cube the tofu, and prepare your baking sheet.

Bake for 25 minutes and allow it to cool.

Combine the sauce ingredients and whisk it thoroughly until you get that well-blended texture. You can add more ingredients, depending on your personal preferences with taste.

Put the tofu in the sauce and stir it quickly to coat the tofu thoroughly. Leave it there for 15 minutes or more for a thorough marinate.

While the tofu marinates, shred the cauliflower into rice- size bits. You can also try buying cauliflower rice from the store to save yourself this step. If you are doing this manually, use a fine grater or a food processor.

Grab a skillet and put it on medium heat. Start cooking the veggies on a bit of sesame oil and just a little bit of soy sauce. Set it aside.

Grab the tofu and put it on the pan. Stir the tofu frequently until it gets that nice golden-brown color. Do not worry if some of the tofu sticks to the pan – it will do that sometimes. Set aside.

Steam your cauliflower rice for 5 to 8 minutes. Add some sauce and stir thoroughly.

Now it is time to add up the ingredients together. Put the cauliflower rice with the veggies and tofu. Serve and enjoy. You can reheat this if there are leftovers but try not to leave it in the fridge for long.

Simple Keto Fried Chicken

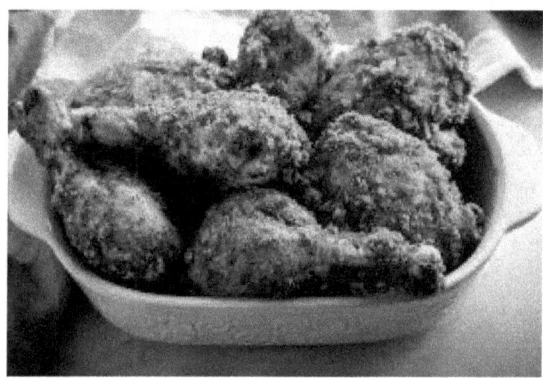

Total time: 45 minutes

Ingredients:

4 boneless and skinless chicken thighs

Frying oil

2 large eggs

2 tbsp. heavy whipping cream

2/3 cup grated parmesan cheese (breading)

2/3 cup blanched almond flour (breading)

1 tsp. salt (breading)

½ tsp. black pepper (breading)

½ tsp. cayenne (breading)

½ tsp. paprika (breading)

Directions:

Grab a bowl and put together the eggs and heavy cream. Beat them together until perfectly mixed.

Grab another bowl, this time combining all the breading ingredients and mix well. Set it aside for now.

Cut the chicken thigh into 3 even pieces. Make sure they are not wet by patting the moist area with a paper towel. This will help prevent the oil splashes when you start frying them.

So now you have the chicken and 2 bowls. One bowl contains the egg wash and the other contains the breading. Dip the chicken in the bread first before dipping it in the egg wash and then finally, dipping it in the breading again. Make sure it is completely covered.

Put 2 inches worth of oil in a pot and heat it up until it reaches around 350 degrees Fahrenheit or when it starts to become steamy. When this happens, try to gradually lower the heat so you can maintain that temperature. This is important since a perfectly heated oil will help create crunchy chicken.

Put the coated chicken in your hot oil. Do this gently with a pair of tongs, making sure there are no splashes of any kind. Frying time should take around 5 minutes or until the coating becomes deep brown in color.

Prepare some paper towels and put the cooked chicken on it. This will help remove any excess oil.

Try not to overcrowd the pan so all of them will cook beautifully. Serve while still crispy for best results.

Keto Butter Chicken

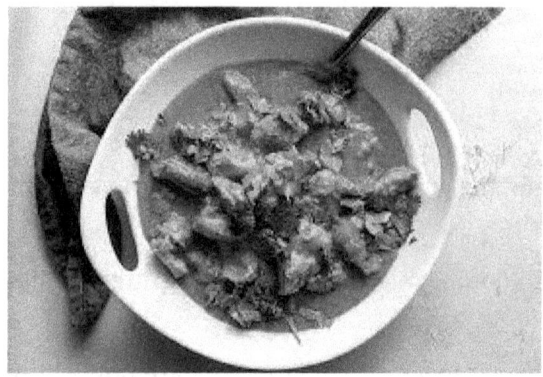

Total time: 35 minutes

Ingredients:

1.5 lb. chicken breast

1 tbsp. coconut oil

2 tbsp. garam masala

3 tsp. grated fresh ginger

3 tsp. minced garlic

4 oz. plain yogurt

2 tbsp. butter (for sauce)

1 tbsp. ground coriander (for sauce)

½ cup heavy cream (for sauce)

½ tbsp. garam masala (for sauce)

2 tsp. fresh ginger, grated (for sauce)

2 tsp. minced garlic (for sauce)

2 tsp. cumin (for sauce)

1 tsp. chili powder (for sauce)

1 onion (for sauce)

14.5 oz. crushed tomatoes (for sauce)

Salt to taste (for sauce)

Directions:

Start by cutting the chicken into pieces measuring around 2 inches each. Place it in a large bowl and add 2 tablespoons of garam masala, 1 teaspoon of minced garlic, and 1 teaspoon of grated ginger. Stir slowly and add the yogurt. Make sure that mix is evenly distributed before putting a lid on the container and chilling it in the fridge for 30 minutes.

For the sauce, grab a blender and put in the ginger, garlic, onion, tomatoes, and spices. Blend until smooth.

Leave the blended sauce aside and grab a skillet. Using medium heat, remove the chicken from the fridge and cook, allowing it to brown on both sides.

Once cooked, pour in the sauce, and allow it to simmer for 5 more minutes

Finally, put in the cream and ghee, still using medium heat. Add some salt for taste and serve!

Keto Shrimp Scampi Recipe

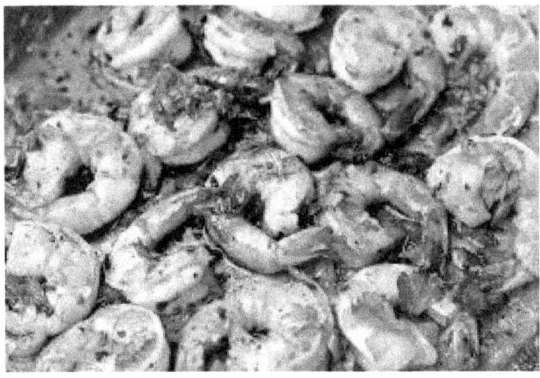

Total time: 35 minutes

Ingredients:

2 summer squash

1-pound shrimp, deveined

2 tbsp. butter unsalted

2 tbsp. lemon juice

2 tbsp. chopped parsley

¼ cup chicken broth

1/8 tsp. red chili flakes

1 clove minced garlic

Salt and pepper to taste

Directions:

Start by cutting the summer squash into noodle-like shapes. You can use a spiralizer to get this done or perhaps use a fork to scrap the surface.

Spread the noodles on top of paper towards and sprinkle them with salt. Set aside for 30 minutes.

Blot the excess water with a paper towel.

In a frying pan, melt butter over medium heat and fry the garlic until you get that fragrant smell. Add some chicken broth, red chili flakes, and lemon juice.

Once it boils, add the shrimp, and allow it to cook. Reduce the heat once the shrimp turns pink.

Add more salt and pepper to taste before adding the summer squash noodles and parsley to the mix. Make sure all the ingredients are well-coated by the sauce. Serve.

Keto Lasagna

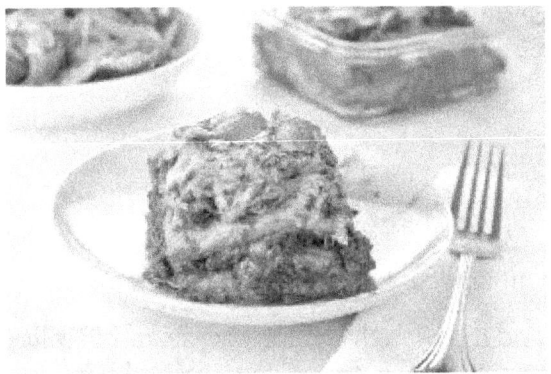

Total time: 1 hour 35 minutes

Ingredients:

8 oz. block of cream cheese

3 large eggs

Kosher salt

Ground black pepper

2 cups of shredded mozzarella

½ cup of freshly grated parmesan

Pinch crushed red pepper flakes

Chopped parsley for garnish

¾ cup marinara (for the sauce)

1 tbsp. tomato paste (for the sauce)

1 lb. ground beef (for the sauce)

½ cup of freshly grated parmesan (for the sauce)

1.5 cup of shredded mozzarella (for the sauce)

1 tbsp. of extra virgin olive oil (for the sauce)

1 tsp. dried oregano (for the sauce)

3 cloves minced garlic (for the sauce)

½ cup chopped onion (for the sauce)

16 oz. ricotta (for the sauce)

Directions:

Start by preheating the oven to 350 degrees and preparing the baking tray by lining it with parchment and cooking spray.

Grab a microwave-safe bowl and throw in the cream cheese, mozzarella, and parmesan, melting them together for a few seconds in the microwave. Mix them in thoroughly before adding the eggs and blending the whole thing together. Add a pinch of salt and pepper for seasoning.

Spread the mixture on a baking sheet and bake for 15 to 20 minutes.

While baking, grab a skillet and using medium heat, coat the surface with oil. Put in the onion and allow them to cook for 5 minutes before adding the garlic. Once you get that fragrant smell, wait 60 more seconds before adding the tomato paste onto the mixture. Make sure to stir all the items around until the onion and garlic are well-coated.

Add the ground beef in the skillet and cook the mixture, breaking up the meat until it is no longer pinks in appearance. Add salt and pepper to taste. Cook it for a few more minutes before setting it aside and allowing it to cool. There should be a bit of fluid remaining in the skillet – try to drain that out of the meat before proceeding with the next step.

Turn on the stove again, keeping the medium heat constant. Add some marinara sauce and season with pepper, red pepper flakes, and ground pepper. Stir around to evenly distribute the flavor.

By this time, your noodles should be ready from the oven. Take them out and start cutting them in half widthwise and then cut them again into 3 pieces.

Start layering! Use an 8-inch baking pan for this, placing 2 noodles at the bottom of the dish first and layer as you wish. Alternate the parmesan and mozzarella shreds depending on your personal preferences.

Bake until the cheese melts and the sauce bubbles out. Should take about 30 minutes.

Garnish and serve.

Creamy Tuscan Garlic Chicken

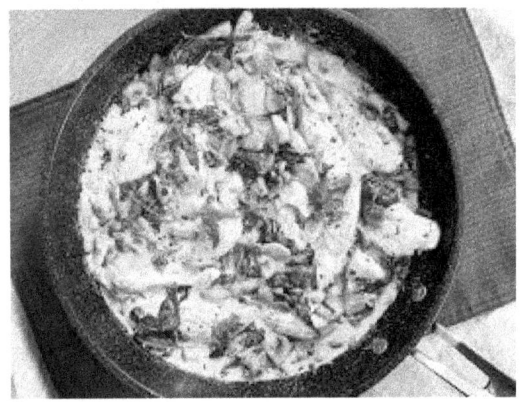

Total time: 30 minutes

Ingredients:

1.5 pounds boneless and skinless chicken breast, thinly sliced

½ cup chicken broth

½ cup parmesan cheese

½ cup sun dried tomatoes

1 cup heavy cream

1 cup chopped spinach

2 tbsp. olive oil

1 tsp. garlic powder

1 tsp. Italian seasoning

Directions:

Grab a large skillet and cook the chicken using olive oil using medium heat. Do this for 5 minutes for each side or until they are thoroughly cooked. Set it aside in a plate.

Using the same skillet, combine the heavy cream, garlic powder, Italian seasoning, parmesan cheese, and chicken broth. Expose it to medium heat and just whisk away until the mixture thickens.

Add the sundried tomatoes and spinach and let it simmer until the spinach wilts.

Add the chicken back and serve.

Bonus method: Fasting

Step 1: Making a Goal

In your journal, write down your goals for fasting. Why do you want to follow the 16/8 method of fasting? Is it to be healthier, to manage medical issues, or just to feel better about your daily life? Have a specific reason for doing the 16/8 method. Having a goal can help keep you motivated to continue fasting, even during difficult times.

Your goal should be a SMART goal. SMART goals are goals that are *specific, measurable, achievable, relevant*, and *time bound*.

Specific. While you might say that your goal is to get healthier in general, this isn't a specific goal. A specific goal is clear and explains exactly where you want to see improvement. Do you want to have better blood sugar levels? Do you want to lose weight or inches from your waistline? Do you want to have more focus during your day? There are a variety of possible specific goals that you can choose from to start your fast.

Measurable. Your goal, whatever it is, should be measurable. There should be measurement that helps you see that you've made improvement. Numbers are a great way to measure your goal's success, but it can also be something beyond numbers, like having a consistent mood. So long as you are tracking your goal and measuring it in some way, your goal will be measurable. If your goal is to have better blood sugar levels, then have a specific number you're aiming for every day. This number can be found by talking with your doctor. If your goal is to lose weight or inches, then have a specific number that you're looking for on the scale or on the measuring tape. If your goal is to have more focus during the day, then track that feeling every day. Many people use mood trackers to help gauge their feelings every day. Trackers like this are perfect for non-tangible goals like feeling more focused, being happier, sleeping better, etc. When you can track your goals, then it is something measurable. If you aren't meeting your goals, you'll see that in your tracking, and you'll know that you need to adjust. And if you are meeting your goals, you can celebrate each milestone and each moment you're closer to fully achieving your goal.

Achievable. Achievable goals are ones that you can reach. If your goal is to lose hundreds of pounds through fasting, that's not quite achievable or realistic. A better goal would be saying you want to lose ten pounds. This is an achievable goal. Once you meet this goal, feel free to create another one where you want to lose another ten pounds. Achievable goals should not be ones that are monumental or ones that are very idealistic. Choose goals that are realistic. We've talked before about how choosing a large goal is not likely to succeed. This is because large goals are often more like a vision far away rather than something that is smaller and doable. Having a large goal can cause your motivation to wane, which is often why people fail at New Year's resolutions. So, choose goals that are achievable. They don't have to be easy; they just must be possible.

Relevant. Let's say that you and your best friend B decide to do the 16/8 method together. This is honestly great because you'll have someone, you're accountable to and someone who supports you. But your goals for the fast should not be the same. Your goals need to be relevant to you. Hugh Jackman did the 16/8 method for preparing his Wolverine role. Does this mean that you should follow his same goals of muscle growth and weight loss? No. He had trainers, nutritionists, and coaches that helped him reach those goals. You probably don't have that support. Besides, are you trying to look like Wolverine? Probably not. Choose goals that are relevant to you personally. Choose the measurements that work for you. Friend B might want to lose 20 pounds, but you might want to just sleep better. So long as the goal is yours, it will be relevant.

Time-bound. Goals that have a specific time to be achieved are beneficial. This doesn't mean that once you've reached your goal, you stop. You can stop if you want to, but you can also repeat the same goal again or make another goal to follow. If your goal is to have better blood sugar levels, when do you want this to happen? If you want to lose weight, when will you achieve this goal? If you want to have more focus at work, at what point will you say you've achieved your goals?

Now that you know what SMART goals are, let's look at a couple of examples of SMART goals. We'll use the examples mentioned above of losing weight, getting better blood sugar levels, and having more focus at work. Here's what a SMART goal might look like:

"I want to lose ten pounds in the next two months through fasting and cooking at home more. I want to fit into my jeans, so I will measure my success by the numbers on the scale and how easily I can slide my jeans over my belly."

This goal is specific because it's clear the person wants to lose weight to fit into their jeans. It's measurable because it has a clear number of ten pounds that can be weighed on a scale. It's achievable because most people can lose ten pounds in two months with changes to their eating schedule and their food. It's also relevant because it's a very personal goal: to fit into their jeans again. Goals don't have to be relevant to anyone else. Just make sure they're relevant to you. Finally, this goal is time-bound, with a deadline of two months. So, this goal is a better-written goal than just saying, "I want to lose weight."

"I want my blood sugar levels after waking up to go down from 150 to 90 points. I want these points to be consistent over the course of two weeks, and I'll achieve this goal in two months by focusing on fasting, my eating habits, and walking 30 minutes every day."

This goal is specific. The person knows exactly what numbers they want to achieve. They probably tested their blood sugar for two weeks after waking up and realized that it was around 150 most or every day. This isn't a healthy blood sugar level after not eating for eight hours. So, they know they want to drop it into a healthy range that is less than 100. The goal is also measurable. We have clear numbers that they can check with a glucose monitor. Having two months to meet this goal makes it achievable, especially through fasting, better eating habits, and exercise. In fact, they may achieve their goal in less time! This goal is relevant to this person because it has specific numbers that they've learned from their own testing. Finally, this goal is time-bound because they have two months to complete it. They also know that the number 90 must be reached for multiple days before they consider the goal to have been met.

"Donna told me that I'm always spacey at work, and I always feel so tired. I want to feel more focused at work by having a less foggy mind and better concentration to work hard. I'll achieve this goal within two months through fasting and having a consistent sleep schedule. I'll also need to feel focused for five consecutive days for me to achieve the goal."

This goal is different from the previous goals because it is something that is intangible. There are no numbers to check. So, this person can measure their goals through a mood tracker that they use every day, or they can keep daily notes in their journal. They may even choose to measure the success of their work projects being completed as a sign of having more focus. Whichever way they choose to measure it, they should write it down as a part of their goal. This goal is achievable and relevant. It gives a very large time frame and fasting with eight hours of sleep can definitely help a person to feel less spacey. Because this person has feedback from others and feels foggy herself, she has a very relevant goal. This goal is also time-bound because this person set two months to achieve more focus, and there is a goal of feeling focused for five consecutive days before the goal is met. So, this goal is a decent SMART goal. All they must do is choose their measurement method for this intangible goal.

By having your goals written down in your journal and having SMART goals, you'll be able to see if intermittent fasting is helping you. You'll also be able to find areas where your goals need to be improved. The journal will help you keep your motivation up.

Step 2: Planning Your Eating Schedule (and Your Sleeping Schedule!)

This is a critical step. You can plan what to eat and where to eat it, but with the 16/8 method, it's all about *when* you eat. Remember, you only have an eight-hour window to eat, so what time will you have breakfast (or will you not have breakfast), what time will you have lunch, and when will you have dinner? Consider things like your current work schedule or family schedule. Do you want to eat dinner right before the beginning of your fasting time, or do you want to eat it a bit earlier? Consider all these factors. If you exercise regularly, you'll want to eat immediately after eating. However, this is just a suggestion. Some people feel weak if they don't eat something before exercising, so choose your schedule based on your feeling. Also, consider special events. How will your schedule change have based on these events? At the end of this chapter, we'll share some example fasting schedules, but be sure to adapt them to your own life.

One thing to consider when making your schedule is following your natural circadian rhythm. We've discussed this in chapter 1, but this is a recommended schedule. It sometimes doesn't work for many people. During your day, your metabolism is often fastest in the morning and slumps around 3:00 p.m. At this point, it begins its slow-down process preparing for the night. So, you can choose to have your eating window from 7:00 a.m. to 3:00 p.m. and eat you meals there, following your circadian rhythm. However, remember that this schedule doesn't work for everyone. It also doesn't give you the opportunity to eat during social events in the evening. While it doesn't give you a social life mealtime, you can always adjust your fasting and eating window to fit a planned event. You don't want to be the only one at the table who is drinking a glass of water while everyone else eats. So, plan when you'll eat to fit your own lifestyle.

It's ideal to follow the 16/8 method daily, and most people do. However, you don't have to! Some people follow it during the workweek but then skip the weekends to better fit in social eating and drinking. Choose whatever will work for you. You can also work with your doctor to help plan out your schedule.

While we're talking about schedules, it's important to also have a consistent sleep schedule. Set a consistent time to go to bed and a consistent time to wake up and follow it. This will help you figure out how many hours you need to fast each day. If you're going to go to bed at 11:00 p.m. and wake up at 7: a.m., then you can fit your fasting schedule around that. You could do your additional eight hours of fasting before you go to bed, or you could divide it into four hours before bed and four hours after you wake up. If you have a consistent sleep time but don't follow it, then it's useless. So, make sure you're following it. If you know it takes you 30 minutes of downtime before you fall asleep, then be in bed 30 minutes earlier, read a book, have some water, and then try to fall asleep at your set time. Use your alarm clock to wake up and don't keep hitting the snooze button. Overall, this consistency will help you better manage your fast.

Step 3: Planning Your Meals

Here comes the science. You need to find meals that will fit in your daily nutrition requirements and calories and keep you full. Consider snacks. Will you snack during your day? How will you break your fast? With a full meal, protein drink, or nothing? All of this should take into consideration your daily activities. If you're exercising, you'll want to make sure you have enough energy to both exercise and not be hungry during the fasting period. You can experiment with meals and then write down the results of those meals in your fasting journal. Did you feel hungry quickly after eating? Then you'll need to change around your meal. If you find that you're craving something, then you might be missing a nutrient in your meal. For example, if you're craving peanut butter, add more protein to your meals. In general, the health department has some good guidelines for how many calories to eat per day. You can then divide these calories into your meals and your snacks (if you choose to snack). All this information below is from health.gov. Because these values are for an "average" adult in height and weight, you'll need to calculate it further based on your own weight and height. You can use various websites to find the right calories for maintaining or losing weight.

Here are your recommended daily calories if you are sedentary, of average height, and average weight provided by health.gov:

Age	Male (5'10", 154 lbs.)	Age	Female (5'4", 126 lbs.)
19–20	2,600	19–25	2,000
21–40	2,400	26–50	1,800

41–60	2,200	46–	1,600
61–	2,000		

Here are your recommended daily calories if you're moderately active, of average height, and average weight:

Age	Male (5'10", 154 lbs.)	Age	Female (5'4", 126 lbs.)
19–25	2,800	19–25	2,200
26–45	2,600	26–50	2,000

46–65	2,400	46–	1,800
66–	2,200		

While these are suggested calories, remember that with intermittent fasting and the 16/8 method, many people end up having unplanned calorie restriction. Much of this is anecdotal, but many people have a hard time eating this many calorie in eight hours. Try to ensure you're getting enough calories in a day with enough nutrition. But if you end up taking in a couple of hundred fewer calories because you simply can't eat that much, that's okay.

Now, you don't have to count calories for this fast. A lot of people like to so that they know their meals will keep them full, but it's not a requirement. So long as you are choosing well-balanced meals that are both plentiful and nutritious, you'll be okay. Don't eat junk for an entire meal because then you'll just be hungry an hour later.

We'll explore more about possible foods and menus for your 16/8 fast in a later chapter.

Step 4: Taking a Before Picture

This isn't really a requirement, but many people find it incredibly motivating. Not only can it motivate you, but you're before picture can motivate others too. If you look at a variety of blogs about people's journeys with fasting, you'll always see a before and after/current picture. This can be really motivating for the person in the picture to see their change. Seeing the physical differences in your body from before and after your fast can make you feel happy. So, take a before picture! Add it to your journal, and as you reach some of your goals, take other pictures to commemorate your success.

Step 5: Sleeping Well the Night before You Start

Now we're getting into starting the fast. The day before you start your new fast, you want to make sure you begin your preparation. Try to sleep well before you start. This will help your body prepare itself and start the process of syncing your circadian rhythm. Remember, it's a process, and you want to start on the right foot. The next day (day 1 of your fast), have a good breakfast. That night, you'll start your fasting hours.

Step 6: Starting the Transition

Start your fast gradually. Don't start by doing all 16 hours at once. Instead, break it down over the course of a couple of weeks. Assuming you sleep for eight hours a night, you only need to fast an additional eight hours during your waking hours. In week 1, for the first three days, stop eating an hour before you go to bed, and start eating one hour after you wake up. This puts you at a 10-hour fast, with 14 hours to eat. After those first three days, you're going to add an hour to before bed and after waking up. So, you'll stop eating two hours before bed and start eating two hours after waking up. This puts you at a 12-hour fast, with 12 hours to eat. Three days later, add another two hours, bringing you up to a 14-hour fast, and a 10-hour eating period. Then finally, extend to the full 16 hours of fasting and 8 hours of eating. This should slowly get you into the full fast and help curb the discomfort you might feel. This will take about two weeks to get to the full fast.

One thing to mention is that exercise should be reduced during this time, and water consumption should be increased. As you get used to the fast, you can increase your exercise, but just at the beginning, you might struggle with exercising with fasting. You should also be drinking a lot more liquid as you transition into the fast. You'll want to keep hydrated because your body will start noticing that there is a larger and larger window of nothing coming in. Have water to keep you hydrated and help curb your appetite if you're feeling hungry during your fasting window.

You are, of course, welcome to just jump in and do the full 16 hours of fasting and 8 hours of eating, but with this jump into fasting, you'll have some discomfort for the first week or so. We'll discuss discomfort in the next step.

Step 7: Preparing Yourself for Magic . . . and Discomfort

While starting your fast, you need to prepare yourself for some changes to your body and habits. You might feel some discomfort with the change. This includes things like strange sleep patterns or dreams, changes in your mood, and sometimes bloating or digestive discomfort. These will usually pass after a couple of weeks of fasting. Some people are lucky and never feel the discomfort, but others do. Take the time to evaluate what you're feeling. If something is feeling way off, stop fasting and talk to your doctor. Signs to stop and talk with your doctor are feelings of weakness and dizziness, changes to your heart rate or respiration, and severe discomfort.

It's very likely that you'll also feel some positive changes within the first week. Many people feel like their brains are clearer. This means that they have more focus and awareness of their environment, with less fogginess. This is a great feeling. It comes with the changes to your hormonal patterns but also the reset to your circadian rhythm. Embrace the change! Within a couple of weeks, you'll notice other changes. In research, after eight weeks of fasting, there were decent metabolic changes that people were able to maintain. This includes changes to blood glucose levels, insulin levels, and other hormones. These changes will make you feel better than you're used to, which is a great benefit that comes with fasting.

Step 8: Recording Your Progress

The final step is to keep track of your progress and record it all in your fasting journal. Note times when your meals didn't work out and times when they did. Also, record times when you felt discomfort and times when you felt fantastic with your fast! Include pictures, little motivational notes—really, anything that will help you keep on track.

Check your journal regularly. This can give you some motivation, but it can also help you find areas to tweak your fast to better fit your life. Your journal is your journey recorded. You can use it to help motivate others but also remind you of the progress you have made. Keep it up and keep recording your progress.

Conclusion

It is hard to know where the truth is if you are just starting to look for a diet that works for you. You have already been sorted out by scientists. The plain truth is you are going to have to educate yourself, weigh the arguments, then follow your own best judgment. My experience has been largely positive, but for one reason or another you will have heard of friends who have problems with low carbohydrate diets. There is no such thing as a miracle diet, and most of them are just variations on a theme, but all keto diets are based on a very specific principle, which has been shown to induce weight loss in many people. You might want to try to base your opinion on the evidence available, not on anecdotes. After all, it is your body and health.

All the best!

Keto diet cookbook for women over 50:

A guide to understand the keto diet for women over 50. with several easy and delicious low-carb recipes.

Introduction

Whatever reason your diet did not work out for, the truth is some diets are simply not feasible. They can be hard to stick to and plan meals around. For those with busy schedules diets that are complex just do not work. Maybe the diet saps all your energy away due to the food changes, or lack of food that you are eating. Maybe it just simply does not work. Who knows? Who cares?

So, why read this book at all then? Maybe you are just curious about Keto or flirting with the idea of trying another diet. Yup, there's that pesky word again. Diet. But Keto is not just a diet or a fad; it is a lifestyle change you will not ever want to get off. There are so many reasons to want to try out the Keto diet.

If you have heard a little bit about the Keto diet, this might not sound so odd to you. If this is your first time really reading about the Keto diet, you might be thinking: "High fat?

I promise if you stick with this guide it will all be revealed to you, and you will be happier and healthier for all the Keto knowledge. There have been extensive studies conducted about the Keto diet that have proven its long-term health benefits.

The Keto diet can drastically improve your life! If your goal is sustained weight loss when you pick this guide up, that is great! That is precisely what the Keto diet can help you achieve. If you have other goals for lowering your risks for some common health diseases, then keep reading; because the Keto diet can help you with that too! If your goal with this diet is just to lead a healthier lifestyle, that is what the Keto diet is all about.

So, put down that bag of chips, (I said high fat, not bad fat) and let us get started! Sometimes information can be overwhelming, especially with all the different websites out there. You never know if what you are learning is genuine. There is so much to learn and explore with the Keto diet that I have created the ultimate guide here that will get you kick started on the journey to better health. This guide will have it all. From explanations to benefits, to risks and even a meal prep plan!

Sometimes people get wary at the idea of a new meal prep plan, but the Keto diet's meal plan is so ridiculously easy. You probably already have half of this stuff in your pantry. The idea behind this diet is not to starve you but to make you conscious of what you are eating. Healthier food choices will lead to a healthier diet, and in turn, having a healthier diet will lead to sustained weight loss. The Keto diet is not a one-shot gimmick where you lose a lot of weight fast, and in five weeks you have gained it all back. This diet aims to help you maintain yourself and keep that weight off.

Although the Keto diet is backed by many experiments and studies that have been performed, and there are thousands of success stories to prove its results I am not a medical doctor. Visit your doctor to make sure the Keto diet is right for you. It is always good to be on the safe side, and let your doctor tell you if the Keto diet is a perfect match. Everything I do show you in this guide is backed by evidence. I hope that through your journey, you become another one of the thousands of Keto successes out there!

Keto for Women Over 50

Women—we go through so much in life, don't we? From growing up, discovering the joys of life, pursuing a promising career, becoming a mother; there is so much that changes within such a short span of time.

While that is a part of life, what anyone would genuinely try and avoid would be the part where we put on excessive weight that we carry around like an unneeded luggage. It is embarrassing, it is distracting, and it is causing quite a few internal issues as well.

If you thought the biggest hurdle you will face when you hit 50 is a big belly, think again. This isn't the only problem we face. While there are those who would say that having a generous belly is the biggest problem, I firmly believe that there are more serious issues to worry about than that. When it comes to women, well things aren't looking good.

Our bodies, since birth, continuously undergo changes. Most of these changes do not harm us and are only natural. However, once we enter into our 50s, things are a lot different. Now, any changes within our body will directly affect how we perform, operate and work. If we were to keep these changes unchecked and pay no close attention, things would take a turn for the worse.

Most of these issues will remain the same for men as well, however, due to the chemistry of our bodies and differences, both internal and external; both would end up facing a variety of issues exclusive to their gender.

There are a few ways we can avoid these issues. Some of these ways require you to go back in time and start working out from a very young age, control your diet, and change your habits. Obviously, that is the stuff of science fiction and hence is out of the equation.

Other ways would include visiting a doctor and getting pills and energy boosters to help us feel better while taking more pills to fight off diabetes, high blood pressure, and other health issues. This way is not just hectic but far too complicated as well.

For a very long time, the only other way was to avoid worrying too much and hope that life would fix issues itself, and that never ended well for many. People were then left with a worry and a gap that nothing was able to fill. In comes ketogenic diet.

Call it a need of the hour, a savior in disguise or anything you like, the fact remains that this is proving to be a popular option that is not only delivering results but is also helping millions to maintain a healthy lifestyle and reverse some of the damage their bodies have suffered.

Numerous studies have gone on to support the idea that Keto diets are far more effective for the older men and women compared to the younger folks. With so much to look forward to and so little to sacrifice, it does make sense to state that Keto is essentially becoming your permanent way of life once you hit 50, but why is that? Why is it that I and so many others are proclaiming Keto as an important lifestyle choice for women above 50? The answer to this involves some explanation, but I will do my best to do just that!

Keto: The Need of the Hour

Calling something the need of the hour is quite a statement. Anyone to claim something being so important must have sufficient material and facts to back such a claim with. While I have provided what exactly Keto does, there is much to be learned and explored of just why Keto is important for women over the age of 50.

So far, we have learned that women over 50 would face issues like:

- Being overweight

- Running low on energy

- Feeling drowsy and lethargic all the time

- Unable to focus on task

- Glucose levels going haywire

- Blood pressure issues

These are the most common ones but dig a little deeper and you quickly realize that these are just the tip of the iceberg that lies hidden in plain sight.

Menopause

There comes an age in a woman's life where her menstrual cycle will finally end. This is a phase that means your ovaries stop releasing eggs, better known as ovulation, and therefore menstruation ends. This condition is generally observed in women above the age of 40. There is no defined age that shows when a woman can expect menopause.

There are times where women may experience menopause prematurely as well. This happens if a woman has undergone surgeries like hysterectomy (surgery that involves removal of ovaries). It can also happen from any injuries that may have caused damage to the ovaries. If this happens before the age of 40, it is classified as premature menopause.

Menopause, as harmless as it sounds, can be quite a troubling phase for women. The hot flashes you experience will keep you up at night, with an elevated heartbeat. The constant feeling of being irritated and a clear downfall in your sex life can contribute greatly towards you feeling more and more grumpy.

Menopause takes a toll on your hormonal balance and the newly developed imbalance then pushes your body to gain massive weight, experience mood swings like never before and a libido that is crashing faster than you can imagine.

If you think this is bad, here are some other issues that menopause can lead to:

- Chronic stress

- Anxiety

- Insulin spike

- Type 2 Diabetes

- Heart Diseases

- Polycystic ovary syndrome (PCOS)

The overall picture, then, is grim! Fortunately, a difference of lifestyle and a carefully thought-out diet plan can change all that for you. I am not saying it happens overnight or within a week, but the profound impacts are felt rather quickly. In the longer run, Keto will rescue you and your body from impending doom and allow you to lead a life without worrying about keeping a glucose monitor or any of the typical health-related equipment near you.

The Keto diet, while there are many classes of it, helps your hormones to remain in shape and balanced. This means that you do not have to worry about the insulin or any other hormones, hence minimizing the hot flashes and other symptoms. Even if they occur, they will be minor and far less painful.

Moreover, the Keto diet jump-starts your sex drive. The fat-rich diet improves fat-soluble vitamins absorption. Not to forget it especially helps with vitamins D, a vital piece that goes missing with age. All in all, this provides all the drive you need to have intimate moments even in your fifties.

Heart Diseases

Keto diets help women over 50 to shed those extra pounds. Reducing any amount of weight greatly reduces the chances of a heart attack or any other heart complications. Through the carefully selected diet routine, not only are you losing weight and enjoying scrumptious meals, but you are significantly boosting your heart's health and reviving yourself from the otherwise dull state that you may have been in before.

Diabetes Control

Needless to say, the careful selection of ingredients, when cooked together, provide rich nutrients, free from any processed or harmful contents such as sugar. Add to that the fact that Keto automatically controls your insulin levels. The result is a glucose level that is always under control and continued control would lead to a day where you will say goodbye to the medications you might be taking for diabetes.

And so Much More!

By taking up the challenge and adapting the Keto way, you are ensuring yourself one of the safest journeys into the older years, if not the safest of the lot. Sure, there will be days where you may miss a food or two, but that craving will be overshadowed by the benefits the Keto diet will bring for you.

With the help of the Keto diet, you can expect a few more benefits such as:

- Improved and stable blood pressure levels

- A deeper sleep for those suffering from insomnia

- Improved kidney function

- More energy that lasts all day

- Improved bodily functions

All Set to Begin?

Great! Let me be the first one to let you know that you are not too late to start. The fact is no one is ever too late to change their eating, sleeping, and working habits. All it takes is a spark of motivation, and if you are reading this line, you already have that spark. All you need now is to grab a pen and a paper to note down some fine recipes and jot down the things you need and the things you should avoid. Better yet, maintain a little diary or a notebook which you can refer to whenever you wish.

Things to Know Before Trying Keto

The meal plan for a Keto diet aims to reduce carbs drastically, according to Kristen Mancinelli, a dietician based in New York and the author of The Ketogenic Diet: A Scientifically Proven Approach to Fast, Healthy Weight Loss, you can begin with an amount of 20 to 30 grams of carbohydrates every day.

You also have to know carb-rich foods, protein and fat. This enables you to choose the foods that will keep you in a ketogenic diet wisely. For example, you may think that only foods such as pasta, cookies, pasta, bread, ice-cream and candy are rich in pasta. Although beans have some proteins, it is a food that is rich in carbohydrates. Also, many vegetables and fruits have high carbohydrate content. Foods that contain little or no carb include pure fats, butter, oils and meat.

Know Your Relationship with Fatty Food

As a woman above 50, this is an important aspect that can't be overlooked. According to Mancinelli, the common belief of many people is that the intake of fat can kill them. Another confusion about this is that there is currently no conclusive result in support or against the belief. According to some researches, eating of poly-unsaturated fats instead of saturated is essential to reduce the risk of heart disease. On the other hand, many other research studies point towards the fact that total fat and various types of fats are not related to cardiovascular diseases. This controversy makes choosing what to eat a little confusing. Despite all these confusions, it is essential to note that as a woman of over 50, the food you eat contains far more than one nutrient. So, what is important is the total quality of the diet, although more research is still needed to determine the risk and health benefit of Keto.

Another factor to take note of is that your body is not what it used to be, considering that you are now older. To prepare your body for a high-fat diet, you have to make little adjustments in your meals. For instance, you can take green vegetables with fries when taking burgers on lettuce leaves. You can take it up a notch and from time to time.

You will begin to let your body know that a Keto diet meal plan is on its way.

In situations where you should take potatoes or rice in your meal, you can instead choose a non-starchy vegetable. When cooking, you can start using more oil such as avocado or olive oil. You will have to do away with old dieting habits. You can't just go to make a grilled plain-looking skinless chicken breast, as this doesn't make sense when on Keto. This is because it doesn't contain enough fat.

It is important that you make up your mind on Keto, as being afraid can hinder it from working. Thereafter, you can slowly push out carbs from your diet.

Change Your View of Protein – Keto Diet Consists of a Moderate Amount of Protein

Many people usually think that Keto diet involves eating as much protein as you can eat. As a woman of over 50, your metabolism is slightly different from when you were younger. On the norm, your diet shouldn't contain a high quantity of protein. Keto doesn't involve just watching only carbs; you have to take a moderate amount of protein. Protein can easily be converted to glucose. As a result, excessive protein intake can ruin your Keto diet. When a large amount of protein is converted to glucose, your body will come out of ketosis. You can think of your diet as a large number of fatty foods that consist of a small amount of protein, rather than the other way around.

Train yourself to be Able to prepare your Keto Meals Because Carb-rich Processed Foods are Not Okay on Keto

You can go through various Keto-approved recipes to find the ones you will love. I recommend finding up to 6 recipes that you like. This way, you will not end up turning to carbs when looking for what to eat. And it also provides you with a range of different options for meals.

Bulletproof Coffee – A Keto-friendly Drink

This is a mixture of butter and coconut oil in your coffee. It is one drink that has been proven to keep people on Keto away from hunger. Thus, it creates and gives you enough time to choose your next meal.

It is essential to know that coconut oil is capable of increasing Low-Density Lipoprotein (LDL), also called bad cholesterol. So, if you are a woman of 50 and predisposed to the heart or cardiovascular diseases due to family history or other factors, you would want to avoid this drink. To be on the safe side, you can take it up with your doctor.

Let Your Family Know About Your Goal for Weight Loss with Dieting

It is essential to tell your family members of your right loss plan. Being on Keto diet might mean a reduced time eating together with them during mealtimes. To prepare them, as well as yourself to your new habit, you need to speak with them. You can assure them that your new habit which will last between three to six months is only temporary.

As an older woman, the support of your family can be very important. They may not like what you are doing very much, but if it helps you to achieve your goal, they will support you. According to a research published in 2014, having the support of families and everyone around you is a massive help to dieters. It helps them to follow through their diets to lose weight. It is also healthy for them throughout their lifetime. It doesn't hurt to let everyone know what you are trying to achieve with your Keto diet. This makes them less likely to suggest treats or any other unfriendly Keto food for you when you are out with them.

Know the Side Effects and What to Expect. For Instance, the Keto Flu

Ketogenic diets have lots of benefits, one of which is that it helps you lose weight. However, for all its benefits, Keto has some significant side effects. One of such is the Keto flu. Keto flu refers to the time your body uses to adjust to using fat as its major source of energy when you begin your Keto diet. Although many people just do fine despite the massive change in diets. Others, on the other hand, can be downright miserable due to the change, thereby needing time to adjust.

During the first 10 to 12 weeks, you might be extremely weak, as your limbs might feel lethargic. It might be really difficult to perform tasks like climbing upstairs. Another symptom is the usual mental fog many people complain of. Some other common side effects include constipation and diarrhea. This is mostly due to the change in fiber.

Because of this adjustment time, if you want to start dieting, you will have to pick a time when you are not swamped with work and crazy deadlines. Pick a time when everything is slow when you can get the rest you need. Also, within the first few weeks, you might want to cut back on some vigorous exercises by taking it easy. This is because your body is getting used to burning more fats instead of carbs as fuel.

Increase Intake of Electrolytes to Combat Side Effects of Keto Diet

When your body is in a state of ketosis, your body excretes a large volume of water and electrolytes. As your body gets older, it finds it more difficult to compensate for various fluctuations in water and electrolyte balance. With the Keto diet, your electrolyte and water balance might come under a lot of stress. So, it is essential to observe the balance. Since your body is in a state of ketosis, you are more likely to lose much water and electrolyte. As a result, you will need to take the right amount of potassium and sodium as well as water to maintain balance. Include salts in your foods, and take things like salted bone broth drinks, vegetables with low carb content- like asparagus bell peppers, arugula and kale.

Know When Keto is Not Right For You

Ketogenic diet is one of the many famous ways of losing weight. There are many hybrid ketogenic diets. One of them is the "ketotarian." It is a ketogenic diet that consists of primary plants with room for ghee, fish, shellfish and eggs. Although this approach is healthy, it is not very advisable to do Keto while a vegan. Your food options as a vegan are significantly limited when on Keto. For instance, because of the high carb content of lentils or beans, some nuts and seeds, you will probably end up with tofu. And in the end, you will rely on low-carb protein powder. This means as a vegan, you might not be successful in achieving your goal with Keto, especially if you want to stay healthy while doing so.

Some medical conditions might make Keto hard for you to do. For instance, women of over 50 years' experience an overall slowdown of metabolic activities. You should at least see your doctor before going on Keto.

Another example is seen in people who take insulin, oral and non-oral, to maintain high blood pressure and sugar. Having GIT problems is another barrier to Keto. This is because constipation is a side effect of Keto. Therefore, going on Keto that includes a relatively low intake of enough fiber is not the best idea for you.

Also, if your current food restrictions include foods such as eggs, dairy, nuts, soy or maybe seafood, going on Keto will limit you even further, which will not be healthy. As a result, going from a state of restrictive diet to another like Keto is not advisable.

Have a Plan After Keto? After All, Keto Isn't a Forever Plan for Weight Loss

Keto diets are not a forever eating plan. It is made to be for a short time, although many people are capable of going through ketogenic diet a few times in a year. However, many others can just use it to lose weight and then get rid of it later.

According to the standard of the American Heart Association, approximately 47 percent of American adults eat diets that are below standard. Older women, it is especially important to eat healthily. Remember, your body is not what it used to be, and any unhealthy eating predisposes you to many diseases. Going on Keto might be a way for you to change those bad habits. There is always the risk of going back to your old ways after you are done with Keto. After Keto, don't just go straight into the standard everyday meal. Doing so might quickly drop you off the wagon and regain some weight.

Benefits of a Low-Carb Diet for Women

When you are following low-carb and low-fat diets, you can reduce your weight effectively, according to a study from the American Association of Retired Persons (AARP). A low-carb diet comes with many health advantages that are worth the lifestyle change. The mentioned study tested the effects of a low-carb diet on knee pain in adults, an issue experienced by 15% of people in the US. After some patients were subjected to a low-fat diet, practitioners realized that making this change in our eating habits has a big impact on reducing knee pain. The authors suggested it could be a substitute for pain-relieving opioids.

In addition, low-carb diets can assist in improving the HDL cholesterol and triglyceride levels compared to the carb-heavy diets, according to a study from the Mayo clinic. This may be because of the nature of the low-carb diet: a lot of proteins, healthy fats, and unprocessed fats. These foods are very healthy, unlike the standard American diet. Nowadays, low-carb diets like the Keto diet, the Paleo diet, and the Mediterranean diet have become very popular. All these diets are based around controlling carbohydrate intake and helping to increase the ingestion of healthy fats.

Low-Carb Diet Essentials

A very low-carb regimen will gradually add carbs as long as the practitioner is still losing weight. Often low-carb diets start by restricting carbohydrates down to 60 grams daily, according to the Mayo clinic. A lot of the carbs that are eaten in the low-carb diet are obtained from vegetables such as the cauliflower and leafy greens.

When you lose weight, most low-carb diets slowly bring back carbohydrates into your meals. Carb cycling is a well-known way a lot of people re-integrate carbs into their diets, according to the Cleveland Clinic. This consists of planning your carb ingestion for the week based on your active and inactive days. Eat foods with slightly more carbs on your active days and eat low carb meals on your inactive days.

Types of Food to Eat on a Low-Carb Diet

To keep your carbs low, east mostly carb-free proteins like pork, beef, turkey, chicken, eggs, and seafood. Cheese also has protein, but most cheese has just one gram of carbohydrates for every ounce. Fiber is very important for women in their 40s because it keeps sugar levels in the bloodstream from hiking up faster, according to a study from the University of California San Francisco Medical Center.

A low-carb diet will make it very difficult to follow dieticians' recommendation of eating 25 grams daily, which makes it necessary to eat a lot of non-starchy veggies. The veggies you should be eating include sprouts, spinach, kale, mushrooms, onions, and lettuce, among many others.

These vegetables have five grams of net carbs or less, and according to Yale Medicine, since they don't boost sugar levels in the bloodstream, they are not included in the net carb count. Fruits also have rich fiber content and carbs that fit in the low-carb plan. Pumpkin, olives, and avocado have very few grams of carbs for every serving.

Soy foods such as the tofu, edamame, and tempeh are low in net carbs, as they have 6 grams on average for every serving. They are also a source of protein and serve as a substitute for meat. Other foods are full of fiber, vitamins, and minerals. You will add flavor to your meals with carb-free fats like olive oil, avocado, or ghee oil. Keep an eye on the salad dressings, because many of them have hidden sugars.

A Sampling of the Low-Carb Meal Plan

If you set 30 grams of carbs in a day for breakfast, you could have a crustless frittata made with eggs, swiss cheese, chopped asparagus, and onions. You can serve it with ham or bacon. You can opt for a lean chicken breast at lunchtime. You may also mix chopped steak, boiled eggs that have been sliced, cucumbers, crumbled bacon, or olive oil dressing. Close your day with nicely cooked broiled salmon and

153

roasted Brussels sprouts. Low-carb snacks include avocado, boiled eggs, celery sticks, olives, and sliced cucumbers.

In case you have carbs to store, add in fiber-rich nuts once in a while. You can use an ounce of pecans, hazelnuts, or almonds consisting of 3 grams of net carbs. Those who want to lose weight should consider calorie count. Nuts are full of nutrition, but are calorie dense snacks; thus, you are advised to ingest the right ratio.

Pros and Cons of the Keto Diet

You may have heard the words "Keto diet" in some interactions. Maybe you saw it in advertising or on social media. You may have seen images of fatty meals like cheese, coffee, butter, or bacon. Like many things, what you see may be different from what is true. The ketogenic diet is very different from other diets, making it truly one of a kind. The high-fat and low-carb ingestion make Keto quite different from other diets.

Ketogenesis can be seen as a new concept, but it's just a natural process your body changes to when it doesn't have enough glucose to be used as energy. This will cause the body to break down fat and manufacture ketones as a source of energy. This is like a backup generator in the body.

Glucose is the main source of energy in your body, and when its levels are low, ketones are made from ketogenesis to produce energy. This substitution of metabolic actions in the body is called ketosis. Your liver has a function to help in the production of the ketones, but the total required changes are based on your car and protein ingestion. The manufacturing of ketones will slow down if they are not needed. When you follow the Keto diet, your body does not have sufficient glucose as fuel. Thus, your body goes into a state of ketosis.

Pros

· Epilepsy: The ketogenic diet was first put on the spotlight as a cure for seizures, and it has been a successful treatment for many years, with the research showing its benefits.

154

· Mass loss: There are a lot of metabolic changes in this diet. Fat oxidation will increase, as the body will adapt to the higher intake of fat. Fat oxidation and reduction of fat in the body are two separate processes. A higher oxidation of fat doesn't mean there is a reduction in body fat. The key determinant in fat reduction will be total calories ingested minus total calories burned.

· Diabetes type 2: When you restrict your carb intake, your glucose concentrations decrease. This can be a very direct way of controlling diabetes. Be sure to consult a specialist before you use this strategy.

· Cancer: There is a vast area of research surrounding the ketogenic diet. One study shows that tumor cells break down glucose faster in comparison to normal cells. This theory shows that when you starve the tumor cells of glucose, cancer cell growth is hindered, which helps in cancer prevention.

Cons

A review from the Harvard School of Public Health suggests there are some side effects that come with prolonged use of the ketogenic diet. This includes the degradation of kidney stones, osteoporosis, and an increase in blood levels of uric acid. Here are the main side effects associated with following the Keto diet:

· Nutrient deficiencies: Keto's restrictions can prevent you from obtaining some of the nutrients found in grains, as well as fruits that are restricted from the diet. Lacking these nutrients can enhance certain diseases. Every food has a nutritional impact; thus, you are supposed to focus on meats, seafood, vegetables, legumes, and fruits to acquire fiber. Consult with dietitians to address any possibility of deficiencies.

· Keto flu: When you have a diet transition, you may experience some uncomfortable effects as a result of cutting carbs. Some call this the Keto Flu. You may have headaches, hunger, nausea, or constipation that lasts for a few days. Sleeping and hydration will help, but they won't have too much of an impact on the diet transition.

·   Adherence: The high-fat component of the diet may be challenging. You may find it hard to be satisfied with the limited variety of foods and groups that do not permit you to eat tasty foods such as some fruit, grains, ice cream, and cream-based groups. The fact is you have to go outside your comfort zone to follow a healthy diet. To get the long-term health benefits, you have to eat healthy all year instead of just 30 days at a time.

·   Gut health: You may have trouble using the restroom because it is hard to remove the whole grain and fruits, which reduce fiber ingestion in the body. This is not great for gut health.

In summary

·   Considering fat loss, you may want to try something provisionally, and if it has a positive impact, you can consider the physical benefits that come with losing fat.

·   A ketogenic diet has some missing food groups, so some vital nutrients are not available.

·   You have to consult a specialist with knowledge of nutrient and diets. This is not just to monitor your scale, but to know what is going on with your body so you have proper guidance.

·   You should always be aware of the need to supply your body with all the nutrients it needs while you are on a diet. A vitamins-packed diet includes high-quality foods that make it easier to withstand the diet despite the fat loss, muscle increase, and overall maintenance.

Challenges Women Over 50 Faces during Keto Diet and How to Avoid Them

Keto diet is quite simple; just eat 75% fats, 20% protein and 5% carbs. It is a general practice most ketogenic beginners follow, and they maintain their body quite quickly. However, when you cross the age of 50, there are many challenges which you have to go through. Below is the list of those challenges along with their solutions.

Keto-flu

An abrupt shift of diet, from the normal intake of carbs to a limited amount, can cause Keto-flu, also known as carb withdrawal. It usually occurs after one to two days of withdrawal. Its symptoms include headache, muscle soreness, poor focus, sugar cravings, brain fog, irritability, insomnia, or weakness. Your body will take some time to switch from burning carbohydrates to burning fats. Therefore, an abrupt transformation of diet sends your body into starvation mode, hence giving you those unpleasant symptoms. Follow the below tips to help you ease discomforts and symptoms of Keto flu.

Stay well hydrated

How much you should drink depends on your body weight. Divide it divide your body weight by 2. The resulting number of ounces is the water you need to drink per day. The best way to add water is by consuming bone broth in your diet. It will provide not only electrolytes such as potassium and sodium to your body but also water.

Electrolytes supplementation

Electrolytes such as sodium, magnesium and potassium are the key players when it comes to getting better and faster results on a Keto diet. If that is not enough in your body, which is usually common if you are on a low carb diet, try incorporating them by taking electrolytes supplements.

Consume more healthy fats

To enhance your adaptation phase, try to eat a lot of high-quality fat such as MCT oils because it travels straight to the liver after digestion as compared to other fats; hence it can be used immediately.

Consume exogenous ketone supplement

Exogenous ketone supplements aid fatigue and elevate energy levels by increasing the ketone levels in the blood. If you opt for this path, go for a smaller dose of these supplements. Take them, especially during the first five days of the Keto flu.

Muscle cramps and dehydration

Carbs need water for their storage, unlike fats. Hence, instead of being retained, a smaller amount of water is stored during the Keto diet, and more amount of sodium is excreted by the kidneys. Due to this, you can easily get dehydrated while on the Keto diet, especially at the beginning. Due to this condition, low electrolyte concentration and dehydration, muscle cramping is certain.

Solution

☐　consult your doctor and complain to him/her about the problems you are facing.

☐　add electrolytes supplements, especially the three major electrolytes such as potassium, sodium and magnesium.

☐　ensure drinking a lot of water in order to remain hydrated; remember the rule of dividing your body weight by 2.

Insomnia

Although, there is not any research which has shown the effect of a Keto diet on sleep deprivation, there some people who have complained about lack of quality sleep during the Keto diet. If this is the case with you, then once in a while eating some high–quality carbs before bed can prove to be of huge help.

Solution

Before sleeping, take one teaspoon of raw honey. This will give your body adequate high-quality carbs during your sleep.

Brain fog

When you eat fewer carbs, your body demands it; "i am hungry, and i want something to eat". When its wish isn't accommodated, it makes you fuzzy headed. This is the brain's way of demanding more glucose. Because, up until now, that's the only fuel it has ever known.

Solution

The best solution to remedy this condition is to ignore it and keep eating fat simply! Ultimately, your brain will adapt to its new fuel, and your head will become clearer than ever before.

Constipation

Consuming carbs lesser than 20g of per day means insufficient fibers, which ultimately results in constipation and irritable bowel syndrome, constipation also occurs when you are not drinking enough water. Following are some remedies to aid you in your constipation.

Solution

☐ add leafy and good vegetables in your diet.

☐ try cyclical Keto from time to time. This will enable you to eat foods like butternut squash and sweet potatoes.

☐ add enough natural salt such as himalayan pink salt in your diet to help you retain water and make your bowels regular.

☐ always remain hydrated and take electrolytes supplements.

☐ do exercise regularly, it will also help you in relieving constipation problems.

☐ try to take the recommended dosage of a good-quality digestive enzyme before or after every meal.

☐ consume psyllium husk every morning. Mix 1 teaspoon in ½ cup of water and let it sit for 1 minute before drinking.

Diarrhea

Some people have diarrhea difficulties while on the Keto diet. Your body may react this way because of an increasing amount of fat intake; as it isn't yet able to produce and store enough bile to break down all the fat, you're eating.

Solution

☐ reduce the amount of fat you're eating by at least 10 per cent.

☐ simultaneously, increase the number of fermented foods in your diets such as kombucha, water kefir, sauerkraut, kimchi, or your favorite fermented vegetable.

☐ add apple cider vinegar to your drinks and salad dressings.

☐ consider trying an ox bile supplement.

☐ to cure diarrhea, lower your fat intake for seven days — or until you are adapted to the new changes. Then, gradually increase your fat intake back up to where it was.

Keto rash

Keto rash also called prurigo pigmentosa is an itchy red rash that can develop on neck, chest, back and armpit areas; it is neither dangerous nor life-threatening. Although very rare, it sometimes occurs when people follow a strict ketogenic diet, usually 80 percent fat or higher. Other causative agents are hormonal imbalances, allergens exposure and gut bacteria.

Solution

☐ support your skin with adequate supplements and anti-inflammatory foods such as dha, omega- 3 supplements, or turmeric latte. This will boost the healing time while soothing the rash.

☐ keep yourself away from irritants like heat, sweat, or friction. Keto rash just like other rashes that can become worse when connecting with irritants. Avoid these irritants by putting on loose and breathable clothes, avoiding scented products or perfumes or any sweat-stimulating exercise until your skin is properly healed.

☐   reintroduce some carbs in your diet; though avoid consuming a lot of bread. However, if rash occurs after a sudden shift to a Keto lifestyle, it is essential for you to bring back some high quality and healthy carbs such as butternut squash, pumpkin, carrots, yams and sweet potatoes.

Breakfast Recipes

Almond Butter Muffins

Preparation Time: 10 minutes

Cooking Time: 25 minutes

Servings: 6

Ingredients:

1cups almond flour

1/2 cup powdered erythritol

1 teaspoons baking powder

¼ teaspoon salt

¾ cup almond butter, warmed

¾ cup unsweetened almond milk

2 large eggs

Directions:

Preheat the oven to 350 ° F, and line a paper liner muffin pan.

In a mixing bowl, whisk the almond flour and the erythritol, baking powder, and salt.

Whisk the almond milk, almond butter, and the eggs together in a separate bowl.

Drop the wet ingredients into the dry until just mixed together.

Spoon the batter into the prepared pan and bake for 22 to 25 minutes until clean comes out the knife inserted in the middle.

Cook the muffins in the pan for 5 minutes. Then, switch onto a cooling rack with wire.

Nutrition:

Calories: 135 kcal

Fat: 11g

Protein: 6g

Carbohydrates: 4g

Fiber: 2g

Net carbs: 2g

Classic Western Omelet

Preparation Time: 5 minutes

Cooking Time: 10 minutes

Servings: 1

Ingredients:

2 teaspoons coconut oil

3 large eggs, whisked

1 tablespoon heavy cream

Salt and pepper

¼ cup diced green pepper

¼ cup diced yellow onion

¼ cup diced ham

Directions:

In a small bowl, whisk the eggs, heavy cream, salt, and pepper.

Heat up 1 teaspoon of coconut oil over medium heat in a small skillet.

Add the peppers and onions, then sauté the ham for 3 to 4 minutes.

Spoon the mixture in a cup and heat the skillet with the remaining oil.

Pour in the whisked eggs and cook until the egg's bottom begins to set.

Tilt the pan and cook until almost set to spread the egg.

Spoon the ham and veggie mixture over half of the omelet and turn over.

Let cook the omelet until the eggs are set and then serve hot.

Nutrition:

Calories: 415 kcal

Fat: 32.5g

Protein: 25g

Carbs: 6.5g

Sugar: 1.5g

Net carbohydrates: 5g

Sheet Pan Eggs with Ham and Pepper Jack

Preparation Time: 5 minutes

Cooking Time: 15 minutes

Servings: 6

Ingredients:

12 large eggs, whisked

Salt and pepper

2 cups diced ham

1 cup shredded pepper jack cheese

Directions:

Preheat the oven to 350°F and grease a rimmed baking sheet with cooking spray.

Whisk the eggs in a mixing bowl then add salt and pepper until frothy.

Stir in the ham and cheese and mix until well combined.

Pour the mixture in baking sheets and spread into an even layer.

Bake for 12 to 15 minutes until the egg is set.

Let cool slightly then cut it into squares to serve.

Nutrition:

Calories: 235 kcal

Fat: 15g

Protein: 21g

Carbs: 2.5g

Fiber: 0.5g

Net carbs: 2g

Tomato Mozzarella Egg Muffins

Preparation Time: 5 minutes

Cooking Time: 25 minutes

Servings: 12

Ingredients:

1 tablespoon butter

1 medium tomato, finely diced

½ cup diced yellow onion

12 large eggs, whisked

½ cup canned coconut milk

¼ cup sliced green onion

Salt and pepper

1 cup shredded mozzarella cheese

Directions:

Preheat the oven to 350 ° F and grease the cooking spray into a muffin pan.

Melt the butter over moderate heat in a medium skillet.

Add the tomato and onions, then cook until softened for 3 to 4 minutes.

Divide the mix between cups of muffins.

Whisk the bacon, coconut milk, green onions, salt, and pepper together and then spoon into the muffin cups.

Sprinkle with cheese until the egg is set, then bake for 15 to 25 minutes.

Nutrition:

Calories: 135 kcal

Fat: 10.5g

Protein: 9g

Carbs: 2g

Fiber: 0.5g

Net carbs: 1.5g

Crispy Chai Waffles

Preparation Time: 10 minutes

Cooking Time: 20 minutes

Servings: 4

Ingredients:

4 large eggs, separated into whites and yolks

3 tablespoons coconut flour

3 tablespoons powdered erythritol

1 ¼ teaspoon baking powder

1 teaspoon vanilla extract

½ teaspoon ground cinnamon

¼ teaspoon ground ginger

Pinch ground cloves

Pinch ground cardamom

3 tablespoons coconut oil, melted

3 tablespoons unsweetened almond milk

Directions:

Divide the eggs into two separate mixing bowls.

Whip the whites of the eggs until stiff peaks develop and then set aside.

Whisk the egg yolks into the other bowl with the coconut flour, erythritol, baking powder, cocoa, cinnamon, cardamom, and cloves.

Pour the melted coconut oil and the almond milk into the second bowl and whisk.

Fold softly in the whites of the egg until you have just combined.

Preheat waffle iron with cooking spray and grease.

Spoon into the iron for about ½ cup of batter

Cook the waffle according to directions from the maker.

Move the waffle to a plate and repeat with the batter left over.

Nutrition:

Calories: 215 kcal

Fat: 17g

Protein: 8g

Carbohydrates: 8g

Fiber: 4g

Net carbs: 4g

Broccoli, Kale, Egg Scramble

Preparation Time: 5 minutes

Cooking Time: 10 minutes

Servings: 1

Ingredients:

2 large eggs, whisked

1 tablespoon heavy cream

Salt and pepper

1 teaspoon coconut oil

1 cup fresh chopped kale

¼ cup frozen broccoli florets, thawed

2 tablespoons grated parmesan cheese

Directions:

In a mug, whisk the eggs along with the heavy cream, salt, and pepper.

Heat 1 teaspoon coconut oil over medium heat in a medium-size skillet.

Stir in the kale and broccoli, then cook about 1 to 2 minutes until the kale is wilted.

Pour in the eggs and cook until just set, stirring occasionally.

Stir in the cheese with parmesan and serve hot.

Nutrition:

Calories: 315 kcal

Fat: 25g

Protein: 19.5g

Carbs: 10g

Fiber: 1.5g

net carbs: 8.5g

Three Cheese Egg Muffins

Preparation Time: 5 minutes

Cooking Time: 20 minutes

Servings: 8

Ingredients:

1 tablespoon butter

½ cup diced yellow onion

12 large eggs, whisked

½ cup canned coconut milk

¼ cup sliced green onion

Salt and pepper

½ cup shredded cheddar cheese

½ cup shredded Swiss cheese

¼ cup grated parmesan cheese

Directions:

Preheat the oven to 350 ° F and grease the cooking spray into a muffin pan.

Melt the butter over moderate heat in a medium skillet.

Add the onions then cook until softened for 3 to 4 minutes.

Divide the mix between cups of muffins.

Whisk the bacon, coconut milk, green onions, salt, and pepper together and then spoon into the muffin cups.

In a cup, mix the three kinds of cheese, and scatter over the egg muffins.

Bake till the egg is set, for 20 to 25 minutes.

Nutrition:

Calories: 150 kcal

Fat: 11.5g

Protein: 10g

Carbs: 2g

Fiber: 0.5g

net carbs: 1.5g

Bacon, Mushroom, and Swiss Omelet

Preparation Time: 5 minutes

Cooking Time: 10 minutes

Servings: 1

Ingredients:

3 large eggs, whisked

1 tablespoon heavy cream

Salt and pepper

2 slices uncooked bacon, chopped

¼ cup diced mushrooms

¼ cup shredded Swiss cheese

Directions:

Whisk the eggs together in a small bowl with heavy cream, salt, and pepper.

Cook the bacon over medium to high heat in a small skillet.

Spoon it in a mug, when the bacon is crisp.

Steam the skillet over medium heat, then add the chestnuts.

Cook the mushrooms until they smoke, then spoon the bacon into the dish.

Heat the skillet with the remaining oil.

Pour in the whisked eggs and cook until the egg's bottom begins to set.

To scatter the egg, tilt the saucepan and cook until almost set.

Spoon the mixture of bacon and mushroom over half of the omelet, then sprinkle with the cheese and fold over.

Let the omelet cook until the eggs have been set and serve hot.

Nutrition:

Calories: 475 kcal

Fat: 36g

Protein: 34g

Carbohydrates: 4g

Fiber: 0.5g

Net carbs: 3.5g

Coco-Cashew Macadamia Muffins

Preparation Time: 10 minutes

Cooking Time: 25 minutes

Servings: 12

Ingredients:

1 ¾ cups almond flour

1 cup powdered erythritol

¼ cup unsweetened cocoa powder

2 teaspoons baking powder

¼ teaspoon salt

¾ cup cashew butter, melted

¾ cup unsweetened almond milk

4 large eggs

¼ cup chopped macadamia nuts

Directions:

Preheat the oven to 350 ° F and use paper liners to line a muffin pan.

In a mixing bowl, whisk the almond flour along with the erythritol, cocoa powder, baking powder, and salt.

Whisk the almond milk, the cashew butter, and the eggs together in a separate bowl.

Move the wet ingredients to the dry when mixed, then insert into the nuts.

Spoon the batter into the prepared pan and bake for 22 to 25 minutes until clean comes out the knife inserted in the middle.

Cook the muffins in the pan for 5 minutes, and then switch onto a cooling rack with wire.

Nutrition:

Calories: 230g

Fat: 20g

Protein: 9g

Carbohydrates: 9g

Fiber: 2.5g

Net carbs: 6.5g

Maple Cranberry Muffins

Preparation Time: 10 minutes

Cooking Time: 20 minutes

Servings: 12

Ingredients:

¾ cups almond flour

¼ cup ground flaxseed

¼ cup powdered erythritol

1 teaspoon baking powder

⅛ teaspoon salt

⅓ cup canned coconut milk

¼ cup coconut oil, melted

3 large eggs

½ cup fresh cranberries

1 teaspoon maple extract

Directions:

Preheat the oven to 350 ° F, and line a paper liner muffin pan.

In a mixing bowl, whisk the almond flour along with the ground flaxseed, erythritol, baking powder, and salt.

Whisk coconut milk, coconut oil, eggs, and maple extract together in a separate bowl.

Move the wet ingredients to the dry until just full, then fold into the cranberries.

Spoon the batter into the prepared pan and bake for 18 to 20 minutes until clean comes out the knife inserted in the center.

Cook the muffins in the pan for 5 minutes, then switch onto a cooling rack with wire.

Nutrition:

Calories: 125g

Fat: 115.g

Protein: 3.5g

Carbs: 3g

Fiber: 1.5g

Carbs: 11.5g

Chocolate Protein Pancakes

Preparation Time: 5 minutes

Cooking Time: 15 minutes

Servings: 6

Ingredients:

1 cup canned coconut milk

¼ cup coconut oil

8 large eggs

2 scoops (40g) egg white protein powder

¼ cup unsweetened cocoa powder

1 teaspoon vanilla extract

Liquid stevia extract, to taste

Directions:

In a food processor, add the coconut milk, coconut oil, and eggs.

Pulse the mixture several times and then add the other ingredients.

Mix until smooth and well–change sweetness to taste.

Heat medium-heat a non-stick skillet

Using about ¼ cup per pancake, spoon in batter

Cook until bubbles form at the batter's surface, then flip carefully.

Let the pancake cook until it browns on the underside.

The leftover batter is moved to a plate to keep warm and repeat.

Nutrition:

Calories: 455g

Fat: 38.5g

Protein 23g

Carbs: 8g

Fiber: 3g

Net carbs: 5g

Lunch Recipes

Cole Slaw Keto Wrap

Preparation Time: 15 minutes

Cooking Time: 0 minutes

Servings: 2

Ingredients:

For the coleslaw

3 cups sliced thin Red Cabbage

0.5 cups, diced Green Onions

0.75 cups Mayo

2 teaspoons Apple Cider Vinegar

0.25 teaspoon Salt

For the wraps and additional filling

16 pieces, stems removed Collard Green

1 pound, cooked & chilled Ground Meat of choice

0.33 cup Alfalfa Sprouts

Directions:

Mix slaw items with a spoon in a large-sized bowl until everything is well-coated.

Place a collard green on a plate and scoop a tablespoon or two of coleslaw on the edge of the leaf. Top it with a scoop of meat and sprouts.

Roll and tuck the sides to keep the filling from spilling.

Once you assemble the wrap, put in your toothpicks in a way that holds the wrap together until you are ready to beat it. Just repeat this with the leftover leaves.

NOTE: we can store these for 4-5 days, and 4 wraps make for 1 serving.

Nutrition:

Net carbs: 4g

Fiber: 2g

Fat: 42g

Protein: 2g

Calories: 409

Keto Chicken Club Lettuce Wrap

Preparation Time: 15 minutes

Cooking Time: 15 minutes

Servings: 1

Ingredients:

1 head of iceberg lettuce with the core and outer leaves removed

1 tbsp. of mayonnaise

6 slices or organic chicken or turkey breast

Bacon (2 cooked strips, halved)

Tomato (just 2 slices)

Directions:

Line your working surface with a large slice of parchment paper.

Layer 6-8 large leaves of lettuce in the center of the paper to make a base of around 9-10 inches.

Spread the mayo in the center and lay with chicken or turkey, bacon, and tomato.

Starting with the end closest to you, roll the wrap like a jelly roll with the parchment paper as your guide. Keep it tight and halfway through, roll tuck in the ends of the wrap.

When it is completely wrapped, roll the rest of the parchment paper around it, and use a knife to cut it in half.

NOTE: This recipe makes one serving, but the wraps will keep for 3-4 days so you can increase the recipe to have some prepped for lunch through the week.

Nutrition:

Net carbs: 4g

Fiber: 2g

Fat: 78g

Protein: 28g

Calories: 837

Keto Broccoli Salad

Preparation Time: 10 minutes

Cooking Time: 0 minutes

Servings: 4-6

Ingredients:

For your salad

2 medium-sized heads, florets chunked Broccoli

2 cups shredded well Red Cabbage

0.5 cups, roasted Sliced Almonds

1 stalk, sliced Green Onions

0.5 cups Raisins

For your orange almond dressing

0.33 cup Orange Juice

0.25 cup Almond Butter

2 tablespoons Coconut Aminos

1; small-sized, chopped finely Shallot

Half-teaspoon Salt

Directions:

Use a food processor to pulse together salt, shallot, amino, nut butter, and OJ. Make sure it is perfectly smooth.

Use a medium-sized bowl to combine other ingredients. Toss it with dressing and serve.

NOTE: This recipe is around 4-6 serving and can keep for up to 5 days.

Nutrition:

Net carbs: 13g

Fiber: 0g

Fat: 94g

Protein: 22g

Calories: 1022

Caribbean Jerk Shrimp with Cauliflower Rice

Preparation Time: 30 minutes

Cooking Time: 40 minutes

Servings: 8

Ingredients:

For the dish

10 ounces, deveined & peeled Large-sized Shrimp

2 tablespoons EVOO

2 tablespoon) Red Wine Vinegar

2 tablespoons Orange Juice

1 tablespoon, packed) Brown Sugar

1 tablespoon Soy Sauce

2 stalks, chopped Green Onions

1 small-sized, seeded & chopped Jalapenos

Jerk Seasoning:

a half-teaspoon Powdered Garlic

a half-teaspoon Powdered Onion

0.25 teaspoon Thyme

a half-teaspoon Paprika

0.125 teaspoons Allspice

0.125 teaspoons Nutmeg

0.25 teaspoon Powdered Cayenne

0.125 teaspoons Salt

Lime Wedges

For the cauliflower rice

1 tablespoon EVOO

1; small-sized, chopped Green Pepper

1; small-sized, seeded & chopped Jalapeno

1 cup, chopped Pineapple

4 cups Cauliflower Rice

1 teaspoon Powdered Garlic

0.25 teaspoon Salt

0.25 teaspoon Pepper

0.125 teaspoons Cinnamon

0.25 cup Orange Juice

1–15 ounce can, drained Red Kidney Beans

2 tablespoons, chopped fresh herb Cilantro
Directions:

Prepare the marinade first by combining all items from the list. Stir in the shrimp; marinade for only 45 minutes.

Prepare the rice now by combining everything to the skillet from that list. Wait to add cilantro until everything else is warmed. After about 10 minutes, add this herb in.

Now, make the skewers by putting the shrimp on the sticks and grill them outside or on the stovetop. They will probably need 5 minutes per side.

Boil the leftover marinade in a small pot over medium-high temperature. After 1 minute, simmer at low heat for only 10 minutes. Spoon this glaze onto the shrimp. Add rice to the bottom of the prep containers, finishing with adding the shrimp and lime wedges.

Nutrition:

Net carbs: 46g

Fiber: 0g

Fat: 12g

Protein: 30g

Calories: 400 kcal

Keto Sheet Pan Chicken and Rainbow Veggies

Preparation Time: 15 minutes

Cooking Time: 25 minutes

Servings: 4

Ingredients:

Nonstick spray

Chicken Breasts (1 pound, boneless & skinless)

Sesame Oil (1 tablespoon)

Soy Sauce (2 tablespoons)

Honey (2 tablespoons)

Red Pepper (2; medium-sized, sliced)

Yellow Pepper (2; medium-sized, sliced)

Carrots (3; medium-sized, sliced)

Broccoli (half-a-head cut up)

2 Red Onions (medium-size and sliced)

EVOO (2 tablespoons)

Pepper & salt (to taste)

Parsley (0.25 cup, fresh herb, chopped)

Directions:

Spray your baking sheet with cooking spray and bring the oven to a temperature of 400-degrees

Put the chicken in the middle of the sheet. Separately, combine the oil and the soy sauce. Brush the mix over the chicken.

Like the image above shows, separate your veggies across the plate. Sprinkle with oil and then toss them gently to ensure they are coated. Finally, spice up with pepper & salt.

Set tray into the oven and cook for around 25 minutes until all is tender and done throughout.

After taking out of the oven, garnish using parsley. Divide everything between those prep containers paired with your favorite greens.

NOTE: This recipe makes 4 servings and will keep for 4-5 days.

Nutrition:

Net carbs: 9g

Fiber: 0g

Fat: 30g

Protein: 30g

Calories: 437kcal

Skinny Bang Bang Zucchini Noodles

Preparation Time: 15 minutes

Cooking Time: 15 minutes

Servings: 4

Ingredients:

For the noodles

4 medium zucchini spiralized

1 tbsp. olive oil

For the sauce

Plain Greek Yogurt (0.25 cup + 2 tablespoons)

Mayo (0.25 cup + 2 tablespoons)

Thai Sweet Chili Sauce (0.25 cup + 2 tablespoons)

Honey (1.5 teaspoons)

Sriracha (1.5 teaspoons)

Lime Juice (2 teaspoons)

Directions:

If you are using any meats for this dish such as chicken or shrimp, cook them first then set aside. Pour the oil into a large-sized skillet at medium temperature. After the oil heats through, stir in the spiraled zucchini noodles. Cook the "noodles" until tender yet still crispy. Remove from the heat, drain, and set at rest for at least 10 minutes.

Combine sauce items together into a large-sized both until perfectly smooth. Give it a taste and adjust as needed. Divide into 4 small containers. Mix your noodles with any meats you cooked and add to meal prep containers.

When you are ready to eat it, heat the noodles, drain any excess water, and mix in sauce.

NOTE: This recipe will keep for 3 days.

Nutrition:

Net carbs: 18g

Fiber: 0g

Fat: 1g

Protein: 9g

Calories: 161g

Keto Caesar Salad

Preparation Time: 15 minutes

Cooking Time: 0 minutes

Servings: 4

Ingredients:

Mayonnaise (1.5 cups)

Apple Cider Vinegar / ACV (3 tablespoons)

Dijon Mustard (1 teaspoon)

Anchovy Filets (4)

Romaine Heart Leaves (24 of them)

Pork Rinds (4 ounces, chopped)

Parmesan (for garnish)

Directions:

Place the mayo with ACV, mustard, and anchovies into a blender and process until smooth and dressing like.

Prepare romaine leaves and pour out dressing across them evenly.

Top with pork rinds and enjoy.

NOTE: Keep the dressing in separate small containers until you are ready to eat a salad. This recipe should keep for 4-5 days.

Nutrition:

Net carbs: 4g

Fiber: 3g

Fat: 86g

Protein: 47g

Calories: 993kcal

Keto Buffalo Chicken Empanadas

Preparation Time: 20 minutes

Cooking Time: 30 minutes

Servings: 6

Ingredients:

For the empanada dough

1 ½ cups of mozzarella cheese

3 oz. of cream cheese

1 whisked egg

2 cups of almond flour

For the buffalo chicken filling

2 cups of cooked shredded chicken

Butter (2 tablespoons, melted)

Hot Sauce (0.33 cup)

Directions:

Bring the oven to a temperature of 425-degrees.

Put the cheese & creamed cheese into a microwave-safe dish. Microwave at 1-minute intervals until completely combined.

Stir the flour and egg into the dish until it is well-combined. Add any additional flour for consistency - until it stops sticking to your fingers.

With another medium-sized bowl, combine the chicken with sauce and set aside.

Cover a flat surface with plastic wrap or parchment paper and sprinkle with almond flour. Spray a rolling pin to avoid sticking and use it to press the dough flat. Make circle shapes out of this dough with a lid, a cup, or a cookie cutter. For excess dough, roll back up and repeat the process.

Portion out a spoonful of filling into these dough circles but keep them only on one half. Fold the other half over to close up into half-moon shapes. Press on the edges to seal them.

Lay on a lightly greased cooking sheet and bake for around 9 minutes until perfectly brown.

NOTE: This recipe prepares 6 servings and can keep for 4-5 days.

 Nutrition:

Net carbs: 20g

Fiber: 0g

Fat: 96g

Protein: 74g

Calories: 1217kcal

Pepperoni and Cheddar Stromboli

Preparation Time: 15 minutes

Cooking Time: 20 minutes

Servings: 3

Ingredients:

Mozzarella Cheese (1.25 cups)

Almond Flour (0.25 cup)

Coconut Flour (3 tablespoons)

Italian Seasoning (1 teaspoon)

Egg (1 large-sized; whisked)

Deli Ham (6 ounces; sliced)

Pepperoni (2 ounces; sliced)

Cheddar Cheese (4 ounces; sliced)

Butter (1 tablespoon, melted)

Salad Greens (6 cups)

Directions:

First things first, bring the oven to a temperature of 400 degrees and prepare a baking tray with some parchment paper.

Use the microwave to melt the mozzarella until it becomes easy to stir.

Mix flours & Italian seasoning in a separate small-sized bowl.

Dump in the melty cheese and stir together with pepper and salt to taste.

Stir in the egg and process the dough with your hands. Pour it onto that prepared baking tray.

Roll out the dough with your hands or a pin. Cut slits that mark out 4 equal rectangles.

Put the ham and cheese onto the dough, then brush with butter and close up, putting the seal end down. Bake for around 17 minutes until well-browned. Slice up and serve.

NOTE: This makes 3 servings and will keep for 2-3 days. It's best served with a small salad.

Nutrition:

Net carbs: 20g

Fiber: 0g

Fat: 13g

Protein: 11g

Calories: 240kcal

Dinner Recipes

Roasted Cornish Hen

Preparation time: 15 minutes

Cooking time: 1 hour

Servings: 8

 Ingredients:

1 tablespoon dried basil, crushed

2 tablespoons lemon pepper

1 tablespoon poultry seasoning

Salt, as required

4 (1½-pound) Cornish game hens, rinsed and dried completely

2 tablespoons olive oil

1 yellow onion, chopped

1 celery stalk, chopped

1 green bell pepper, seeded and chopped

Directions:

Preheat your oven to 375°F. Arrange lightly greased racks in 2 large roasting pans.

In a bowl, mix well basil, lemon pepper, poultry seasoning, and salt.

Coat each hen with oil and then, rub evenly with the seasoning mixture.

In a next bowl, mix together the onion, celery, and bell pepper.

Stuff the cavity of each hen loosely with veggie mixture.

Arrange the hens into prepared roasting pans, keeping plenty of space between them.

Roast for about 60 minutes or until the juices run clear.

Remove the hens from oven and place onto a cutting board.

With a foil piece, cover each hen loosely for about 10 minutes before carving.

Cut into desired size pieces and serve.

Nutrition:

Calories 714

Net Carbs 2.8 g

Total Fat 52.2 g

Saturated Fat 0.5g

Cholesterol 349 mg

Sodium 235 mg

Total Carbs 3.8 g

Fiber 1 g

Sugar 1.4 g

Protein 58.2 g

Butter Chicken

Preparation time: 15 minutes

Cooking time: 28 minutes

Servings: 5

Ingredients:

3 tablespoons unsalted butter

1 medium yellow onion, chopped

2 garlic cloves, minced

1 teaspoon fresh ginger, minced

1½ pounds grass-fed chicken breasts, cut into ¾-inch chunks

2 tomatoes, chopped finely

1 tablespoon garam masala

1 teaspoon red chili powder

1 teaspoon ground cumin

Salt and ground black pepper, as required

1 cup heavy cream

2 tablespoons fresh cilantro, chopped

Directions:

Melt butter in a large wok over medium-high heat and sauté the onions for about 5–6 minutes.

Now, add in ginger and garlic and sauté for about 1 minute.

Add the tomatoes and cook for about 2–3 minutes, crushing with the back of spoon.

Stir in the chicken spices, salt, and black pepper, and cook for about 6–8 minutes or until desired doneness of the chicken.

Stir in the heavy cream and cook for about 8–10 more minutes, stirring occasionally.

Garnish with fresh cilantro and serve hot.

Nutrition:

Calories 507

Net Carbs 4 g

Total Fat 33.4 g

Saturated Fat 18.6 g

Cholesterol 203 mg

Sodium 211 mg

Total Carbs 5.5 g

Fiber 1.5 g

Sugar 2.3 g

Protein 40.5 g

Chicken & Broccoli Casserole

Preparation time: 15 minutes

Cooking time: 35 minutes

Servings: 6

Ingredients

2 tablespoons butter

¼ cup cooked bacon, crumbled

2½ cups cheddar cheese, shredded and divided

4 ounces cream cheese, softened

¼ cup heavy whipping cream

½ pack ranch seasoning mix

2/3 cup homemade chicken broth

1½ cups small broccoli florets

2 cups cooked grass-fed chicken breast, shredded

Directions:

Preheat your oven to 350°F.

Arrange a rack in the upper portion of the oven.

For chicken mixture: In a large wok, melt the butter over low heat.

Add the bacon, ½ cup of cheddar cheese, cream cheese, heavy whipping cream, ranch seasoning, and broth, and with a wire whisk, beat until well combined.

Cook for about 5 minutes, stirring frequently.

Meanwhile, in a microwave-safe dish, place the broccoli and microwave until desired tenderness is achieved.

In the wok, add the chicken and broccoli and mix until well combined.

Remove from the heat and transfer the mixture into a casserole dish.

Top the chicken mixture with the remaining cheddar cheese.

Bake for about 25 minutes.

Now, set the oven to broiler.

Broil the chicken mixture for about 2–3 minutes or until cheese is bubbly.

Serve hot.

Nutrition:

Calories 449

Net Carbs 2.3 g

Total Fat 33.5 g

Saturated Fat 20.1 g

Cholesterol 133 mg

Sodium 1001 mg

Total Carbs 2.9 g

Fiber 0.6 g

Sugar 0.8 g

Protein 31.3 g

Turkey Chili

Preparation time: 15 minutes

Cooking time: 2¼ hours

Servings: 8

Ingredients

2 tablespoons olive oil

1 small yellow onion, chopped

1 green bell pepper, seeded and chopped

4 garlic cloves, minced

1 jalapeño pepper, chopped

1 teaspoon dried thyme, crushed

2 tablespoons red chili powder

1 tablespoon ground cumin

2 pounds lean ground turkey

2 cups fresh tomatoes, chopped finely

2 ounces sugar-free tomato paste

2 cups homemade chicken broth

1 cup water

Salt and ground black pepper, as required

1 cup cheddar cheese, shredded

Directions:

In a large Dutch oven, heat oil over medium heat and sauté the onion and bell pepper for about 5–7 minutes.

Add the garlic, jalapeño pepper, thyme, and spices and sauté for about 1 minute.

Add the turkey and cook for about 4–5 minutes.

Stir in the tomatoes, tomato paste, and cacao powder, and cook for about 2 minutes.

Add in the broth and water and bring to a boil.

Now, reduce the heat to low and simmer, covered for about 2 hours.

Add in salt and black pepper and remove from the heat.

Top with cheddar cheese and serve hot.

Nutrition:

Calories 234

Net Carbs 4.8 g

Total Fat 12.6 g

Saturated Fat 3.2 g

Cholesterol 81 mg

Sodium 328 mg

Total Carbs 6.9 g

Fiber 2.1 g

Sugar 3.2 g

Protein 24.9 g

Beef Curry

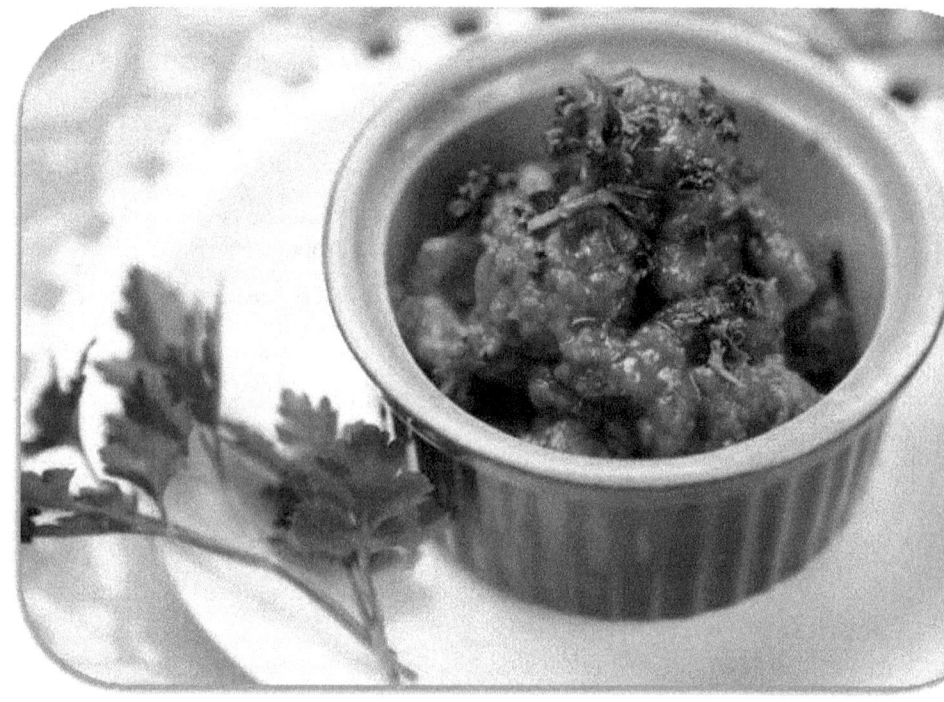

Preparation time: 10 minutes

Cooking time: 3¼ hours

Servings: 8

Ingredients

2 tablespoons butter

2 tomatoes, chopped finely

2 tablespoons curry powder

2½ cups unsweetened coconut milk

½ cup homemade chicken broth

2½ pounds grass-fed beef chuck roast, cubed into 1-inch size

Salt and ground black pepper, as required

¼ cup fresh cilantro, chopped

Directions:

Melt butter in a large pan over low heat and cook the tomatoes and curry powder for about 3–4 minutes, crushing the tomatoes with the back of spoon.

Stir in the coconut milk, and broth, and bring to a gentle simmer, stirring occasionally.

Simmer for about 4–5 minutes.

Stir in beef and bring to a boil over medium heat.

Adjust the heat to low and cook, covered for about 2½ hours, stirring occasionally

Remove from heat and with a slotted spoon, transfer the beef into a bowl.

Set the pan of curry aside for about 10 minutes.

With a slotted spoon, remove the fats from top of curry.

Return the pan over medium heat.

Stir in the cooked beef and bring to a gentle simmer.

Adjust the heat to low and cook, uncovered for about 30 minutes or until desired thickness.

Stir in salt and black pepper and remove from the heat.

Garnish with fresh cilantro and serve hot.

Nutrition:

Calories 666

Net Carbs 3.2 g

Total Fat 53 g

Saturated Fat 27 g

Cholesterol 154 mg

Sodium 204 mg

Total Carbs 4.1 g

Fiber 0.9 g

Sugar 2.8 g

Protein 38.8 g

Shepherd's Pie

Preparation time: 20 minutes

Cooking time: 50 minutes

Servings: 6

Ingredients

¼ cup olive oil

1-pound grass-fed ground beef

½ cup celery, chopped

¼ cup yellow onion, chopped

3 garlic cloves, minced

1 cup tomatoes, chopped

2 (12-ounce) packages riced cauliflower, cooked and well drained

1 cup cheddar cheese, shredded

¼ cup Parmesan cheese, shredded

1 cup heavy cream

1 teaspoon dried thyme

Directions:

Preheat your oven to 350°F.

Heat oil in a large nonstick wok over medium heat and cook the ground beef, celery, onions, and garlic for about 8–10 minutes.

Remove from the heat and drain the excess grease.

Immediately stir in the tomatoes.

Transfer mixture into a 10x7-inch casserole dish evenly.

In a food processor, add the cauliflower, cheeses, cream, and thyme, and pulse until a mashed potatoes-like mixture is formed.

Spread the cauliflower mixture over the meat in the casserole dish evenly.

Bake for about 35–40 minutes.

Remove casserole dish from oven and let it cool slightly before serving.

Cut into desired sized pieces and serve.

Nutrition:

Calories 404

Net Carbs 5.7 g

Total Fat 30.5 g

Saturated Fat 13.4 g

Cholesterol 100 mg

Sodium 274 mg

Total Carbs 9.2 g

Fiber 3.5 g

Sugar 4 g

Protein 24.5 g

Meatballs Curry

Preparation time: 15 minutes

Cooking time: 25 minutes

Servings: 6

Ingredients

Meatballs

1-pound lean ground pork

2 organic eggs, beaten

3 tablespoons yellow onion, finely chopped

¼ cup fresh parsley leaves, chopped

¼ teaspoon fresh ginger, minced

2 garlic cloves, minced

1 jalapeño pepper, seeded and finely chopped

1 teaspoon granulated erythritol

1 teaspoon curry powder

3 tablespoons olive oil

Curry

1 yellow onion, chopped

Salt, as required

2 garlic cloves, minced

¼ teaspoon fresh ginger, minced

1 tablespoon curry powder

1 (14-ounce) can unsweetened coconut milk

Ground black pepper, as required

¼ cup fresh parsley, minced

Directions:

For meatballs: Place all the ingredients (except oil) in a large bowl and mix until well combined.

Make small-sized balls from the mixture.

Heat the oil in a large wok over medium heat and cook meatballs for about 3–5 minutes or until golden-brown from all sides.

Transfer the meatballs into a bowl.

For curry: In the same wok, add onion and a pinch of salt, and sauté for about 4–5 minutes.

Add the garlic and ginger, and sauté for about 1 minute.

Add the curry powder and sauté for about 1–2 minutes.

Add coconut milk and meatballs and bring to a gentle simmer.

Adjust the heat to low and simmer, covered for about 10–12 minutes.

Season with salt and black pepper and remove from the heat.

Top with parsley and serve.

Nutrition:

Calories 350

Net Carbs 4.2 g

Total Fat 29.1 g

Saturated Fat 9.7 g

Cholesterol 55 mg

Sodium 73 mg

Total Carbs 5.2 g

Fiber 1 g

Sugar 2.7 g

Protein 16.2 g

Pork with Veggies

Preparation time: 15 minutes

Cooking time: 15 minutes

Servings: 5

Ingredients

1-pound pork loin, cut into thin strips

2 tablespoons olive oil, divided

1 teaspoon garlic, minced

1 teaspoon fresh ginger, minced

2 tablespoons low-sodium soy sauce

1 tablespoon fresh lemon juice

1 teaspoon sesame oil

1 tablespoon granulated erythritol

1 teaspoon arrowroot starch

10 ounces broccoli florets

1 carrot, peeled and sliced

1 large red bell pepper, seeded and cut into strips

2 scallions, cut into 2-inch pieces

Directions:

In a bowl, mix well pork strips, ½ tablespoon of olive oil, garlic, and ginger.

For sauce: Add the soy sauce, lemon juice, sesame oil, Swerve, and arrowroot starch in a small bowl and mix well.

Heat the remaining olive oil in a large nonstick wok over high heat and sear the pork strips for about 3–4 minutes or until cooked through.

With a slotted spoon, transfer the pork into a bowl.

In the same wok, add the carrot and cook for about 2–3 minutes.

Add the broccoli, bell pepper, and scallion, and cook, covered for about 1–2 minutes.

Stir the cooked pork, sauce, and stir fry, and cook for about 3–5 minutes or until desired doneness, stirring occasionally.

Remove from the heat and serve.

Nutrition:

Calories 315

Net Carbs 5.7 g

Total Fat 19.4 g

Saturated Fat 5.7 g

Cholesterol 73 mg

Sodium 438 mg

Total Carbs 8.3 g

Fiber 2.6 g

Sugar 3 g

Protein 27.4 g

Seafood Recipes

Keto Baked Salmon with Lemon and Butter

Preparation Time: 10 minutes

Cooking Time: 30 minutes

Servings: 3

Ingredients:

1-pound salmon

1 lemon

3 oz. butter

1 tablespoon olive oil

Ground black pepper and sea salt to taste

Directions:

Grease a large-sized baking dish with the olive oil and preheat your oven to 400°F.

Place the salmon on the baking dish, preferably skin-side down. Generously season with pepper and salt to taste.

Thinly slice the lemon and place the slices over the salmon. Cover the fish with ½ of the butter, preferably in very thin slices.

Bake until the salmon flakes easily with a fork and is opaque, for 25 to 30 minutes, on middle rack.

Now, over moderate heat in a small saucepan; heat the remaining butter until it begins to bubble. Immediately remove the pan from heat; set aside and let cool a bit. Gently add in some of the freshly squeezed lemon juice.

Serve the cooked fish with some of the prepared lemon butter and enjoy.

Nutrition:

Calories: 576

Total Fat: 46g

Saturated Fat: 22g

Total Carbohydrates: 1.3g

Dietary Fiber: 0.4g

Sugars: 0.4g

Protein: 31g

Ketogenic Spicy Oyster

Preparation Time: 10 minutes

Cooking Time: 5 minutes

Servings: 2

Ingredients:

12 oysters shucked

1 tablespoon olive oil

7-8 basil leaves, fresh

1 tablespoon garlic chili paste

1/8 teaspoon salt

Directions:

Combine olive oil with garlic chili paste and salt in a medium size mixing bowl; mix well.

Add oysters into the prepared sauce; turning them several times until thoroughly coated.

Create a bed for the oysters to cook by spreading the basil leaves out on an oven-safe dish.

Transfer the oysters and sauce over the bed of basil leaves; spreading them in a single layer on the dish.

Turn on the broiler over high heat.

Place the dish on top rack (approximately a few inches away from the broiler) and broil for a few minutes.

Once done; immediately remove them from the oven. Serve hot and enjoy.

Nutrition:

Calories: 102 kcal

Total Fat: 8g

Saturated Fat: 2.5g

Total Carbohydrates: 2g

Dietary Fiber: 0g

Sugars: 0.3g

Protein: 4g

Garlic Lime Mahi-Mahi

Preparation Time: 15 minutes

Cooking Time: 10 minutes + 30 minutes marinate

Servings: 4

Ingredients:

4 Mahi-Mahi filets (approximately 1 to 1 ¼ pounds)

Zest and juice of 1 large lime, fresh

¼ cup avocado oil

3 cloves garlic, minced

1/8 teaspoon each of ground black pepper and fine grain sea salt

Directions:

For Marinade: Thoroughly combine the entire ingredients (except the filets) together in a small-sized mixing bowl. Pour the mixture on top of filets in a large zip-lock bag or large shallow dish. Let marinate for 30 minutes, at room temperature.

Pour the marinade into a large sauté pan (preferably with a cover) and heat it over medium heat. Once hot; carefully add the filets into the hot pan; cover and cook the filets for a couple of minutes, until cooked through.

Immediately remove the sauté pan from heat; set aside and let rest for 5 minutes, covered. Serve warm and enjoy.

Nutrition:

Calories: 248 kcal

Total Fat: 14g

Saturated Fat: 1.7g

Total Carbohydrates: 0.7g

Dietary Fiber: 0.1g

Sugars: 0g

Protein: 24g

Fish and Leek Sauté

Preparation Time: 15 minutes

Cooking Time: 10 minutes

Servings: 2

Ingredients:

1 leek, chopped

2 trout fillets, diced (approximately 8 oz.)

1 tablespoon tamari soy sauce

1 teaspoon ginger, grated

1 tablespoon avocado oil

Salt to taste

Directions:

Over moderate heat in a large skillet; heat the avocado oil until hot. Once done; add and sauté the chopped leek for a few minutes, until turn soften.

Immediately add the diced trout with grated ginger, tamari sauce and salt to taste.

Continue to sauté the trout until it's not translucent anymore and cooked through.

Serve immediately and enjoy.

Nutrition:

Calories: 175 kcal

Total Fat: 7.6g

Saturated Fat: 1.5g

Total Carbohydrates: 5.2g

Dietary Fiber: 0.8g

Sugars: 1.7g

Protein: 21g

Smoked Salmon Salad

Preparation Time: 5 minutes

Cooking Time: 0 minutes

Servings: 1

Ingredients:

2 oz. smoked salmon

1 lemon slice

4 olives

1 teaspoon pink peppercorns, crushed lightly

A handful of arugula salad leaves, fresh

Directions:

Place the olives and salad leaves into a large plate or shallow bowl.

Arrange the smoked salmon over the salad.

Sprinkle the top of smoked salmon with lightly crushed pink peppercorns.

Garnish your salad with a lemon slice; serve immediately and enjoy.

Nutrition:

Calories: 149 kcal

Total Fat: 5.2g

Saturated Fat: 1.4g

Total Carbohydrates: 4g

Dietary Fiber: 1.7g

Sugars: 3.4g

Protein: 11g

Keto Baked Salmon with Pesto

Preparation Time: 10 minutes

Cooking Time: 30 minutes

Servings: 2

Ingredients:

1 oz. green pesto

½ pound salmon

Pepper and salt to taste

For Green sauce:

¼ cup Greek yogurt

1 oz. green pesto

¼ teaspoon garlic

Pepper and salt to taste

Directions:

Preheat your oven to 400°F.

Arrange the salmon in a well-greased baking dish, preferably skin-side down. Spread the pesto over the salmon and then, sprinkle with pepper and salt to taste.

Bake in the preheated oven until the salmon flakes easily with a fork, for 25 to 30 minutes.

In the meantime, stir the entire sauce ingredients together in a large bowl. Serve the cooked fish with some of the prepared sauce and enjoy.

Nutrition:

Calories: 274 kcal

Total Fat: 21g

Saturated Fat: 3.9g

Total Carbohydrates: 2.9g

Dietary Fiber: 0.6g

Sugars: 1.7g

Protein: 26g

Roasted Salmon with Parmesan Dill Crust

Preparation Time: 10 minutes

Cooking Time: 10 minutes

Servings: 2

Ingredients:

½ pound salmon; cut into pieces

1 tablespoon dill weed

¼ cup cottage cheese

1 tablespoon olive oil

¼ cup parmesan cheese, grated

Directions:

Preheat your oven to 450°F.

Combine cottage cheese with parmesan cheese, olive oil and dill in a large-sized mixing bowl; mix well.

Line a large-sized baking sheet with aluminum foil and then, arrange the salmon pieces on it.

Smear ½ of the cottage cheese mix over the salmon.

Roast in the preheated oven until the fish flakes easily and crust is brown, for 10 minutes.

Serve the cooked fish with the remaining prepared sauce and enjoy.

Nutrition:

Calories: 352 kcal

Total Fat: 22g

Saturated Fat: 6.6g

Total Carbohydrates: 5.7g

Dietary Fiber: 1.5g

Sugars: 0.5g

Protein: 33g

Keto Fried Salmon with Broccoli and Cheese

Preparation Time: 15 minutes

Cooking Time: 25 minutes

Servings: 3

Ingredients:

¾ pound salmon; cut into pieces

3 tablespoons butter

½ pound broccoli; cut into small florets

2 oz. cheddar cheese, grated

Pepper and salt to taste

1 lime

Directions:

Preheat your oven using the broiler settings, to 400°F.

Let the broccoli florets to simmer for a couple of minutes, preferably in lightly salted water. Ensure that the broccoli maintains its delicate color and chewy texture; drain well.

Now arrange the broccoli in a baking dish, preferably well-greased. Add butter and pepper to taste.

Sprinkle with cheese and bake in the preheated oven until the cheese turns golden in color, for 15 to 20 minutes.

Now, over moderate heat in a large saucepan; heat the butter until completely melted and fry the salmon pieces for a couple of minutes per side. Serve the pan-fried salmon with baked broccoli and enjoy.

Nutrition:

Calories: 392g

Total Fat: 25g

Saturated Fat: 11.8g

Total Carbohydrates: 5.8g

Dietary Fiber: 3.4g

Sugars: 1.4g

Protein: 31g

Meat Recipes

Classic Pork Tenderloin

Preparation Time: 15 minutes

Cooking Time: 35 minutes

Servings: 4

Ingredients:

8 bacon slices

2 lb. pork tenderloin

1 tsp. dried oregano, crushed

1 tsp. dried basil, crushed

1 tbsp. garlic powder

1 tsp. seasoned salt

3 tbsp. butter

Directions:

Preheat the oven to 400 degrees F.

Heat a large ovenproof skillet over medium-high heat and cook the bacon for about 6-7 minutes.

Transfer the bacon onto a paper towel lined plate to drain.

Then, wrap the pork tenderloin with bacon slices and secure with toothpicks.

With a sharp knife, slice the tenderloin between each bacon slice to make a medallion.

In a bowl, mix together the dried herbs, garlic powder and seasoned salt.

Now, coat the medallion with herb mixture.

With a paper towel, wipe out the skillet.

In the same skillet, melt the butter over medium-high heat and cook the pork medallion for about 4 minutes per side.

Now, transfer the skillet into the oven.

Roast for about 17-20 minutes.

Remove the wok from oven and let it cool slightly before cutting.

Cut the tenderloin into desired size slices and serve.

Nutrition:

Calories per serving: 471;

Carbohydrates: 1g;

Protein: 53.5g;

Fat: 26.6g;

Sugar: 0.1g;

Sodium: 1100mg;

Fiber: 0.2g

Signature Italian Pork Dish

Preparation Time: 15 minutes

Cooking Time: 15 minutes

Servings: 6

Ingredients:

2 lb. pork tenderloins, cut into 1½-inch pieces

¼ C. almond flour

1 tsp. garlic salt

Freshly ground black pepper, to taste

2 tbsp. butter

½ C. homemade chicken broth

1/3 C. balsamic vinegar

1 tbsp. capers

2 tsp. fresh lemon zest, grated finely

Directions:

In a large bowl, add the pork pieces, flour, garlic salt and black pepper and toss to coat well.

Remove pork pieces from bowl and shake off excess flour mixture.

In a large skillet, melt the butter over medium-high heat and cook the pork pieces for about 2-3 minutes per side.

Add broth and vinegar and bring to a gentle boil.

Reduce the heat to medium and simmer for about 3-4 minutes.

With a slotted spoon, transfer the pork pieces onto a plate.

In the same skillet, add the capers and lemon zest and simmer for about 3-5 minutes or until desired thickness of sauce.

Pour sauce over pork pieces and serve.

Nutrition:

Calories per serving: 373;

Carbohydrates: 1.8g;

 Protein: 46.7g;

Fat: 18.6g;

Sugar: 0.4g;

Sodium: 231mg;

Fiber: 0.7g

Flavor Packed Pork Loin

Preparation Time: 15 minutes

Cooking Time: 1 hour

Servings: 6

Ingredients:

1/3 C. low-sodium soy sauce

¼ C. fresh lemon juice

2 tsp. fresh lemon zest, grated

1 tbsp. fresh thyme, finely chopped

2 tbsp. fresh ginger, grated

2 garlic cloves, chopped finely

2 tbsp. Erythritol

Freshly ground black pepper, to taste

½ tsp. cayenne pepper

2 lb. boneless pork loin

Directions:

For pork marinade: in a large baking dish, add all the ingredients except pork loin and mix until well combined.

Add the pork loin and coat with the marinade generously.

Refrigerate for about 24 hours.

Preheat the oven to 400 degrees F.

Remove the pork loin from marinade and arrange into a baking dish.

Cover the baking dish and bake for about 1 hour.

Remove from the oven and place the pork loin onto a cutting board.

With a piece of foil, cover each loin for at least 10 minutes before slicing.

With a sharp knife, cut the pork loin into desired size slices and serve.

Nutrition:

Calories per serving: 230;

Carbohydrates: 3.2g;

Protein: 40.8g;

Fat: 5.6g;

Sugar: 1.2g;

Sodium: 871mg;

Fiber: 0.6g

Spiced Pork Tenderloin

Preparation Time: 15 minutes

Cooking Time: 18 minutes

Servings: 6

Ingredients:

2 tsp. fresh rosemary, minced

2 tsp. fennel seeds

2 tsp. coriander seeds

2 tsp. caraway seeds

1 tsp. cumin seeds

1 bay leaf

Salt and freshly ground black pepper, to taste

2 tbsp. fresh dill, chopped

2 (1-lb.) pork tenderloins, trimmed

Directions:

For spice rub: in a spice grinder, add the seeds and bay leaf and grind until finely powdered.

Add the salt and black pepper and mix.

In a small bowl, reserve 2 tbsp. of spice rub.

In another small bowl, mix together the remaining spice rub, and dill.

Place 1 tenderloin over a piece of plastic wrap.

With a sharp knife, slice through the meat to within ½-inch of the opposite side.

Now, open the tenderloin like a book.

Cover with another plastic wrap and with a meat pounder, gently pound into ½-inch thickness.

Repeat with the remaining tenderloin.

Remove the plastic wrap and spread half of the dill mixture over the center of each tenderloin.

Roll each tenderloin like a cylinder.

With a kitchen string, tightly tie each roll at several places.

Rub each roll with the reserved spice rub generously.

With 1 plastic wrap, wrap each roll and refrigerate for at least 4-6 hours.

Preheat the grill to medium-high heat. Grease the grill grate.

Remove the plastic wrap from tenderloins.

Place tenderloins onto the grill and cook for about 14-18 minutes, flipping occasionally.

Remove from the grill and place tenderloins onto a cutting board and with a piece of foil, cover each tenderloin for at least 5-10 minutes before slicing.

With a sharp knife, cut the tenderloins into desired size slices and serve.

Nutrition:

Calories per serving: 313;

Carbohydrates: 1.4g;

Protein: 45.7g;

Fat: 12.6g;

Sugar: 0g;

Sodium: 127mg;

Fiber: 0.7g

Sticky Pork Ribs

Preparation Time: 15 minutes

Cooking Time: 2 hours 34 minutes

Servings: 9

Ingredients:

¼ C. Erythritol

1 tbsp. garlic powder

1 tbsp. paprika

½ tsp. red chili powder

4 lb. pork ribs, membrane removed

Salt and freshly ground black pepper, to taste

1½ tsp. liquid smoke

1½ C. sugar-free BBQ sauce

Directions:

Preheat the oven to 300 degrees F. Line a large baking sheet with 2 layers of foil, shiny side out.

In a bowl, add the Erythritol, garlic powder, paprika and chili powder and mix well.

Season the ribs with salt and black pepper and then, coat with the liquid smoke.

Now, rub the ribs with the Erythritol mixture.

Arrange the ribs onto the prepared baking sheet, meaty side down.

Arrange 2 layers of foil on top of ribs and then, roll and crimp edges tightly.

Bake for about 2-2½ hours or until desired doneness.

Remove the baking sheet from oven and place the ribs onto a cutting board.

Now, set the oven to broiler.

With a sharp knife, cut the ribs into serving sized portions and evenly coat with the barbecue sauce.

Arrange the ribs onto a broiler pan, bony side up.

Broil for about 1-2 minutes per side.

Remove from the oven and serve hot.

Nutrition:

Calories per serving: 530;

Carbohydrates: 2.8g;

Protein: 60.4g;

Fat: 40.3g;

 Sugar: 0.4g;

Sodium: 306mg;

Fiber: 0.5g

Valentine's Day Dinner

Preparation Time: 15 minutes

Cooking Time: 35 minutes

Servings: 4

Ingredients:

1 tbsp. olive oil

4 large boneless rib pork chops

1 tsp. salt

1 C. cremini mushrooms, chopped roughly

3 tbsp. yellow onion, chopped finely

2 tbsp. fresh rosemary, chopped

1/3 C. homemade chicken broth

1 tbsp. Dijon mustard

1 tbsp. unsalted butter

2/3 C. heavy cream

2 tbsp. sour cream

Directions:

Heat the oil in a large skillet over medium heat and sear the chops with the salt for about 3-4 minutes or until browned completely.

With a slotted spoon, transfer the pork chops onto a plate and set aside.

In the same skillet, add the mushrooms, onion and rosemary and sauté for about 3 minutes.

Stir in the cooked chops, broth and bring to a boil.

Reduce the heat to low and cook, covered for about 20 minutes.

With a slotted spoon, transfer the pork chops onto a plate and set aside.

In the skillet, stir in the butter until melted.

Add the heavy cream and sour cream and stir until smooth.

Stir in the cooked pork chops and cook for about 2-3 minutes or until heated completely.

Serve hot.

Nutrition:

Calories per serving: 400;

Carbohydrates: 3.6g;

 Protein: 46.3g;

Fat: 21.6g;

Sugar: 0.8g;

Sodium: 820mg;

Fiber: 1.1g

South East Asian Steak Platter

Preparation Time: 15 minutes

Cooking Time: 20 minutes

Servings: 4

Ingredients:

14 oz. grass-fed sirloin steak, trimmed and cut into thin strips

Freshly ground black pepper, to taste

2 tbsp. olive oil, divided

1 small yellow onion, chopped

2 garlic cloves, minced

1 Serrano pepper, seeded and chopped finely

3 C. broccoli florets

3 tbsp. low-sodium soy sauce

2 tbsp. fresh lime juice

Directions:

Season steak with black pepper.

In a large skillet, heat 1 tbsp. of the oil over medium heat and cook the steak for about 6-8 minutes or until browned from all sides.

Transfer the steak onto a plate.

In the same skillet, heat the remaining oil and sauté onion for about 3-4 minutes.

Add the garlic and Serrano pepper and sauté for about 1 minute.

Add broccoli and stir fry for about 2-3 minutes.

Stir in cooked beef, soy sauce and lime juice and cook for about 3-4 minutes.

Serve hot.

Nutrition:

Calories per serving: 282;

Carbohydrates: 7.6g;

Protein: 33.1g;

Fat: 13.5g;

Sugar: 2.7g;

Sodium: 749mg;

Fiber: 2.3g

Pesto Flavored Steak

Preparation Time: 15 minutes

Cooking Time: 17 minutes

Servings: 4

Ingredients:

¼ C. fresh oregano, chopped

1½ tbsp. garlic, minced

1 tbsp. fresh lemon peel, grated

½ tsp. red pepper flakes, crushed

Salt and freshly ground black pepper, to taste

1 lb. (1-inch thick) grass-fed boneless beef top sirloin steak

1 C. pesto

¼ C. feta cheese, crumbled

Directions:

Preheat the gas grill to medium heat. Lightly, grease the grill grate.

In a bowl, add the oregano, garlic, lemon peel, red pepper flakes, salt and black pepper and mix well.

Rub the garlic mixture onto the steak evenly.

Place the steak onto the grill and cook, covered for about 12-17 minutes, flipping occasionally.

Remove from the grill and place the steak onto a cutting board for about 5 minutes.

With a sharp knife, cut the steak into desired sized slices.

Divide the steak slices and pesto onto serving plates and serve with the topping of the feta cheese.

Nutrition:

Calories per serving: 226;

Carbohydrates: 6.8g;

Protein: 40.5g;

Fat: 7.6g;

Sugar: 0.7g;

Sodium: 579mg;

Fiber: 2.2g

Flawless Grilled Steak

Preparation Time: 21 minutes

Cooking Time: 10 minutes

Servings: 5

Ingredients:

½ tsp. dried thyme, crushed

½ tsp. dried oregano, crushed

1 tsp. red chili powder

½ tsp. ground cumin

¼ tsp. garlic powder

Salt and freshly ground black pepper, to taste

1½ lb. grass-fed flank steak, trimmed

¼ C. Monterrey Jack cheese, crumbled

Directions:

In a large bowl, add the dried herbs and spices and mix well.

Add the steaks and rub with mixture generously.

Set aside for about 15-20 minutes.

Preheat the grill to medium heat. Grease the grill grate.

Place the steak onto the grill over medium coals and cook for about 17-21 minutes, flipping once halfway through.

Remove the steak from grill and place onto a cutting board for about 10 minutes before slicing.

With a sharp knife, cut the steak into desired sized slices.

Top with the cheese and serve.

Nutrition:

Calories per serving: 271;

Carbohydrates: 0.7g;

Protein: 38.3g;

Fat: 11.8g;

Sugar: 0.1g;

Sodium: 119mg;

Fiber: 0.3g

Veggie Recipes

Salad Sandwiches

Preparation Time: 5 minutes

Cooking Time: 0 minutes

Servings: 2

Ingredients

1 medium avocado, peeled, pitted, diced

2 leaves of iceberg lettuce

1-ounce unsalted butter

2-ounce cheddar cheese, sliced

Directions:

Rinse the lettuce leaves, pat dry with a paper towel, and then smear each leaf with butter.

Top lettuce with cheese and avocado and Serve and enjoy!

Nutrition:

Calories: 187g

Fats: 17 g

Protein: 5 g

Net Carb: 4 g

Fiber: 1.5 g

Celeriac Stuffed Avocado

Preparation Time: 10 minutes

Cooking Time: 0 minutes

Servings: 2

Ingredients

1 avocado

1 celery root, finely chopped

2 tbsp. mayonnaise

½ of a lemon, juiced, zested

2 tbsp. mayonnaise

Others:

¼ tsp. salt

Directions:

Prepare avocado and for this, cut avocado in half and then remove its pit.

Place remaining ingredients in a bowl, stir well until combined and evenly stuff this mixture into avocado halves.

Serve and enjoy!

Nutrition:

Calories: 285

Fats: 27 g

Protein: 2.8 g

Net Carb: 4.4 g

Fiber: 2.6 g

Cobb salad

Preparation Time: 5 minutes

Cooking Time: 10 minutes

Servings: 1

Ingredients

1 large egg, hard-boiled, peeled, diced

2 oz. chicken thigh

2 1/2 slices bacon, cooked, crumbled

½ of a medium avocado, diced

½ cup chopped lettuce

Others:

1 cup of water

3 tbsp. apple cider vinegar

1 ½ tbsp. coconut oil

¼ tsp. salt

1/8 tsp. ground black pepper

Directions:

Cook chicken thigh and for this, place chicken thighs in an instant pot, pour in 1 cup water, and shut the pot with a lid.

Cook the chicken for 5 minutes at high pressure, and when done, let the pressure release naturally.

Meanwhile, cook the bacon and for this, take a skillet pan, place it over medium heat and when hot, add bacon slices.

Cook the bacon for 3 to 5 minutes until golden brown, then transfer them to a cutting board and chop the bacon, reserve the bacon grease in the pan for the next meal.

When chicken thigh has cooked, transfer it to a bowl and shred the chicken with two forks, reserving the chicken broth for later use.

Assemble the salad and for this, place lettuce in a salad plate, top with chicken, bacon, diced eggs, avocado, and chicken in horizontal rows.

Prepare the dressing and for this, whisk together salt, black pepper, vinegar, and oil until incorporated and then drizzle the dressing generously over the salad.

Serve and enjoy!

Nutrition:

Calories: 206

Fats: 11.8 g

Protein: 19.2 g

Net Carb: 6 g

Fiber: 3 g

Cabbage Hash Browns

Preparation Time: 10 minutes

Cooking Time: 12 minutes

Servings: 2

Ingredients

1 ½ cup shredded cabbage

2 slices of bacon

1/2 tsp. garlic powder

1 egg

Others:

1 tbsp. coconut oil

½ tsp. salt

1/8 tsp. ground black pepper

Directions:

Crack the egg in a bowl, add garlic powder, black pepper, and salt, whisk well, then add cabbage, toss until well mixed and shape the mixture into four patties.

Take a large skillet pan, place it over medium heat, add oil and when hot, add patties in it and cook for 3 minutes per side until golden brown.

Transfer hash browns to a plate, then add bacon into the pan and cook for 5 minutes until crispy.

Serve hash browns with bacon.

Nutrition:

Calories: 336

Fats: 29.5 g

Protein: 16 g

Net Carb: 0.9 g

Fiber: 0.8 g

Cauliflower Hash Browns

Preparation Time: 10 minutes

Cooking Time: 18 minutes

Servings: 2

Ingredients

¾ cup grated cauliflower

2 slices of bacon

1/2 tsp. garlic powder

1 large egg white

Others:

1 tbsp. coconut oil

½ tsp. salt

1/8 tsp. ground black pepper

Directions:

Place grated cauliflower in a heatproof bowl, cover with plastic wrap, poke some holes in it with a fork and then microwave for 3 minutes until tender.

Let steamed cauliflower cool for 10 minutes, then wrap in a cheesecloth and squeeze well to drain moisture as much as possible.

Crack the egg in a bowl, add garlic powder, black pepper, and salt, whisk well, then add cauliflower, and toss until well mixed and sticky mixture comes together.

Take a large skillet pan, place it over medium heat, add oil and when hot, drop cauliflower mixture on it, press lightly to form hash brown patties, and cook for 3 to 4 minutes per side until browned.

Transfer hash browns to a plate, then add bacon into the pan and cook for 5 minutes until crispy.

Serve hash browns with bacon.

Nutrition:

Calories: 347.8

Fats: 31 g

Protein: 15.6 g

Net Carb: 1.2 g

Fiber: 0.5 g

Asparagus, With Bacon and Eggs

Preparation Time: 5 minutes

Cooking Time: 12 minutes

Servings: 2

Ingredients

4 oz. asparagus

2 slices of bacon, diced

1 egg

Others:

¼ tsp. salt

1/8 tsp. ground black pepper

Directions:

Take a skillet pan, place it over medium heat, add bacon, and cook for 4 minutes until crispy.

Transfer cooked bacon to a plate, then add asparagus into the pan and cook for 5 minutes until tender-crisp.

Crack the egg over the cooked asparagus, season with salt and black pepper, then switch heat to medium-low level and cook for 2 minutes until egg white has set.

Chop the cooked bacon slices, sprinkle over egg and asparagus and Serve and enjoy!

Nutrition:

179 Calories;

15.3 g Fats;

9 g Protein;

0.7 g Net Carb;

0.6 g Fiber;

Bell Pepper Eggs

Preparation Time: 10 minutes

Cooking Time: 4 minutes

Servings: 2

Ingredients

1 green bell pepper,

2 eggs

Others:

1 tsp. coconut oil

¼ tsp. salt

¼ tsp. ground black pepper

Directions:

Prepare pepper rings, and for this, cut out two slices from the pepper, about ¼-inch, and reserve remaining bell pepper for later use.

Take a skillet pan, place it over medium heat, grease it with oil, place pepper rings in it, and then crack an egg into each ring.

Season eggs with salt and black pepper, cook for 4 minutes or until eggs have cooked to the desired level.

Transfer eggs to a plate and Serve and enjoy!

Nutrition:

110.5 Calories;

8 g Fats;

7.2 g Protein;

1.7 g Net Carb;

1.1 g Fiber;

Omelet-Stuffed Peppers

Preparation Time: 5 minutes

Cooking Time: 20 minutes

Servings: 2

Ingredients

1 large green bell pepper, halved, cored

2 eggs

2 slices of bacon, chopped, cooked

2 tbsp. grated parmesan cheese

Others:

1/3 tsp. salt

¼ tsp. ground black pepper

Directions:

Turn on the oven, then set it to 400 degrees F, and let preheat.

Then take a baking dish, pour in 1 tbsp. water, place bell pepper halved in it, cut side up, and bake for 5 minutes.

Meanwhile, crack eggs in a bowl, add chopped bacon and cheese, season with salt and black pepper, and whisk until combined.

After 5 minutes of baking time, remove baking dish from the oven, evenly fill the peppers with egg mixture and continue baking for 15 to 20 minutes until eggs has set.

Serve and enjoy!

Nutrition:

428 Calories;

35.2 g Fats;

23.5 g Protein;

2.8 g Net Carb;

1.5 g Fiber;

Bacon Avocado Bombs

Preparation Time: 10 minutes

Cooking Time: 10 minutes

Servings: 2

Ingredients

1 avocado, halved, pitted

4 slices of bacon

2 tbsp. grated parmesan cheese

Directions:

Turn on the oven and broiler and let it preheat.

Meanwhile, prepare the avocado and for that, cut it in half, then remove its pit, and then peel the skin.

Evenly one half of the avocado with cheese, replace with the other half of avocado and then wrap avocado with bacon slices.

Take a baking sheet, line it with aluminum foil, place wrapped avocado on it, and broil for 5 minutes per side, flipping carefully with tong halfway.

When done, cut each avocado in half crosswise and serve

Nutrition:

378 Calories

33.6 g Fats

15.1 g Protein

0.5 g Net Carb

2.3 g Fiber;

Egg in a Hole with Eggplant

Preparation Time: 5 minutes

Cooking Time: 15 minutes

Servings: 2

Ingredients

1 large eggplant

2 eggs

1 tbsp. coconut oil, melted

1 tsp. unsalted butter

2 tbsp. chopped green onions

Others:

¾ tsp. ground black pepper

¾ tsp. salt

Directions:

Set the grill and let it preheat at the high setting.

Meanwhile, prepare the eggplant, and for this, cut two slices from eggplant, about 1-inch thick, and reserve the remaining eggplant for later use.

Brush slices of eggplant with oil, season with salt on both sides, then place the slices on grill and cook for 3 to 4 minutes per side.

Transfer grilled eggplant to a cutting board, let it cool for 5 minutes and then make a home in the center of each slice by using a cookie cutter.

Take a frying pan, place it over medium heat, add butter and when it melts, add eggplant slices in it and crack an egg into its each hole.

Let the eggs cook for 3 to 4 minutes, then carefully flip the eggplant slice and continue cooking for 3 minutes until the egg has thoroughly cooked.

Season egg with salt and black pepper, transfer them to a plate, then garnish with green onions and Serve and enjoy!

Nutrition:

184 Calories

14.1 g Fats

7.8 g Protein

3 g Net Carb

3.5 g Fiber;

Frittata with Spinach and Meat

Preparation Time: 10 minutes

Cooking time: 20 minutes

Servings: 2

Ingredients

4 oz. ground turkey

3 oz. of spinach leaves

1/3 tsp. minced garlic

1/3 tsp. coconut oil

2 eggs

Others:

1/3 tsp. salt

¼ tsp. ground black pepper

Directions:

Turn on the oven, then set it to 400 degrees F, and let it preheat.

Meanwhile, take a skillet pan, place it over medium heat, and add spinach and cook for 3 to 5 minutes until spinach leaves have wilted remove the pan from heat.

Take a small heatproof skillet pan, place it over medium heat, add ground turkey and cook for 5 minutes until thoroughly cooked.

Then add spinach, season with salt and black pepper, stir well, then remove the pan from heat and spread the mixture evenly in the pan.

Crack eggs in a bowl, season with salt and black pepper, then pour this mixture over spinach mixture in the pan and bake for 10 to 15 minutes until frittata has thoroughly cooked and the top is golden brown.

When done, let frittata rest in the pan for 5 minutes, then cut it into slices and Serve and enjoy!

Nutrition:

166 Calories;

13 g Fats;

10 g Protein;

0.5 g Net Carb;

0.5 g Fiber;

Soup Recipes

Cream Zucchini Soup

Preparation Time: 8-10 minutes

Cooking Time: 8 minutes

Servings: 4

Ingredients:

2 cups vegetable stock

2 garlic cloves, crushed

1 tablespoon butter

4 (preferably medium size) zucchinis, peeled and chopped

1 small onion, chopped

2 cups heavy cream

1/2 teaspoon dried oregano, (finely ground)

1/2 teaspoon black pepper, (finely ground)

1 teaspoon dried parsley, (finely ground)

1 teaspoon of sea salt

Lemon juice (optional)

Directions:

Arrange Instant Pot over a dry platform in your kitchen. Open its top lid and switch it on.

Find and press "SAUTE" cooking function; add the butter in it and allow it to melt.

In the pot, add the onions, zucchini, and garlic; cook (while stirring) until turns translucent and softened for around 2-3 minutes.

Add the vegetable broth and sprinkle with salt, oregano, pepper, and parsley; gently stir to mix well.

Close the lid to create a locked chamber; make sure that safety valve is in locking position.

Find and press "MANUAL" cooking function; timer to 5 minutes with default "HIGH" pressure mode.

Allow the pressure to build to cook the ingredients.

After cooking time is over press "CANCEL" setting. Find and press "QPR" cooking function. This setting is for quick release of inside pressure.

Slowly open the lid, take out the cooked recipe in serving plates or serving bowls, and enjoy the Keto recipe. Top with some lemon juice.

Nutrition:

Calories: 490;

Carbohydrates: 11g;

Protein: 23g;

Fat: 6g;

Sugar: 2.2g;

Sodium: 564mg;

Fiber: 1.7g

Coconut Chicken Soup

Preparation Time: 10 minutes

Cooking Time: 18 minutes

Servings: 4

Ingredients:

4 cloves of garlic, minced

1-pound chicken breasts, skin-on

4 cups of water

2 tablespoons olive oil

1 onion, diced

1 cup of coconut milk

(Finely ground) black pepper and salt as per taste preference

2 tablespoons sesame oil

Directions:

Arrange Instant Pot over a dry platform in your kitchen. Open its top lid and switch it on.

Find and press "SAUTE" cooking function; add the oil in it and allow it to heat.

In the pot, add the onions, garlic; cook (while stirring) until turns translucent and softened for around 1-2 minutes.

Stir in the chicken breasts; stir and cook for 2 more minutes.

Pour in water and coconut milk — season to taste.

Close the lid to create a locked chamber; make sure that safety valve is in locking position.

Find and press "MANUAL" cooking function; timer to 15 minutes with default "HIGH" pressure mode.

Allow the pressure to build to cook the ingredients.

After cooking time is over press "CANCEL" setting. Find and press "NPR" cooking function. This setting is for the natural release of inside pressure and it takes around 10 minutes to release pressure slowly.

Slowly open the lid, Drizzle with sesame oil on top.

Take out the cooked recipe in serving plates or serving bowls and enjoy the Keto recipe.

Nutrition:

Calories: 328;

Carbohydrates: 6g;

Protein: 21g;

Fat: 0g;

Sugar: 6g;

Sodium: 609mg;

Fiber: 2g

Chicken Bacon Soup

Preparation Time: 10 minutes

Cooking Time: 40 minutes

Servings: 4

Ingredients:

6 boneless, skinless chicken thighs make cubes

½ cup chopped celery

4 minced garlic cloves

6-ounce mushrooms, sliced

½ cup chopped onion

8-ounce softened cream cheese

¼ cup softened butter

1 teaspoon dried thyme

Salt and (finely ground) black pepper, as per taste preference

2 cups chopped spinach

8 ounces cooked bacon slices, chopped

3 cups (preferably homemade) chicken broth

1 cup heavy cream

Directions:

Arrange Instant Pot over a dry platform in your kitchen. Open its top lid and switch it on.

Add the ingredients except for the cream, spinach, and bacon; gently stir to mix well.

Close the lid to create a locked chamber; make sure that safety valve is in locking position.

Find and press "SOUP" cooking function; timer to 30 minutes with default "HIGH" pressure mode.

Allow the pressure to build to cook the ingredients.

After cooking time is over press "CANCEL" setting, find and press "NPR" cooking function. This setting is for the natural release of inside pressure and it takes around 10 minutes to release pressure slowly.

Slowly open the lid, stir in cream and spinach.

Take out the cooked recipe in serving plates or serving bowls and enjoy the Keto recipe. Top with the bacon.

Nutrition:

Calories: 490;

Carbohydrates: 7g;

Protein: 23g;

Fat: 6g;

Sugar: 2.2g;

Sodium: 742mg;

Fiber: 1.7g

Cream Pepper Soup

Preparation Time: 8-10 minutes

Cooking Time: 10 minutes

Servings: 4

Ingredients:

1 (preferably medium size) celery stalk, chopped

1 (preferably medium size) yellow bell pepper, chopped

1 (preferably medium size) green bell pepper, chopped

2 large red bell peppers, chopped

1 small red onion, chopped

2 tablespoons butter

1/2 cup cream cheese, full fat

1/4 teaspoon dried thyme, (finely ground)

1/2 teaspoon black pepper, (finely ground)

1 teaspoon dried parsley, (finely ground)

1 teaspoon salt

2 cups vegetable stock

1 cup heavy cream

Directions:

Arrange Instant Pot over a dry platform in your kitchen. Open its top lid and switch it on.

Find and press "SAUTE" cooking function; add the butter in it and allow it to heat.

In the pot, add the onions, bell pepper, and celery; cook (while stirring) until turns translucent and softened for around 3-4 minutes.

Pour in the vegetable stock and heavy cream — season with salt, pepper, parsley, and thyme.

Close the lid to create a locked chamber; make sure that safety valve is in locking position.

Find and press "MANUAL" cooking function; timer to 6 minutes with default "HIGH" pressure mode.

Allow the pressure to build to cook the ingredients.

After cooking time is over press "CANCEL" setting, find and press "QPR" cooking function. This setting is for quick release of inside pressure.

Slowly open the lid, mix in the cream; take out the cooked recipe in serving plates or serving bowls, and enjoy the Keto recipe.

Nutrition:

Calories: 286;

Carbohydrates: 9g;

Protein: 4g;

Fat: 0g;

Sugar: 2g;

Sodium: 445mg;

Fiber: 0g

Ham Asparagus Soup

Preparation Time: 10 minutes

Cooking Time: 55 minutes

Servings: 4

Ingredients:

5 crushed garlic cloves

1 cup chopped ham

4 cups (preferably homemade) chicken broth

2 pounds trimmed and halved asparagus spears

2 tablespoons butter

1 chopped yellow onion

½ teaspoon dried thyme

Salt and freshly (finely ground) black pepper, as per taste preference

Directions:

Arrange Instant Pot over a dry platform in your kitchen. Open its top lid and switch it on.

Find and press "SAUTE" cooking function; add the butter in it and allow it to heat.

In the pot, add the onions; cook (while stirring) until turns translucent and softened for around 4-5 minutes.

Add the garlic, ham bone and broth; stir, and cook for about 2-3 minutes.

Add the other ingredients; gently stir to mix well.

Close the lid to create a locked chamber; make sure that safety valve is in locking position.

Find and press "SOUP" cooking function; timer to 45 minutes with default "HIGH" pressure mode.

Allow the pressure to build to cook the ingredients.

After cooking time is over press "CANCEL" setting, find and press "QPR" cooking function. This setting is for quick release of inside pressure.

Slowly open the lid, add the prepared recipe mix in a blender or processor.

Blend or process to make a smooth mix. Place the mix in serving bowls and enjoy the Keto recipe.

Nutrition:

Calories: 146;

Carbohydrates: 5g;

Protein: 29.4g;

Fat: 6g;

Sugar: 2.2g;

Sodium: 222mg;

Fiber: 4g

Beef Zoodle Soup

Preparation Time: 5 minutes

Cooking Time: 13 minutes

Servings: 4

Ingredients:

4 tablespoons Avocado oil

3 tablespoons Minced ginger

1 tablespoon Minced garlic

1 ½ pound Sirloin steak tips, cut into 1-inch pieces

2 cups Broccoli florets

8 ounces Bella mushrooms, sliced

6 cups Beef broth

1/4 cup Apple cider vinegar

1/4 cup Coconut aminos

1/4 cup Sriracha sauce

1 large zucchini, spiralized into noodles

Directions:

Switch on the instant pot, grease pot with oil, press the 'sauté/simmer' button, wait until the oil is hot and add the steak pieces along with ginger and garlic.

Cook steak for 5 minutes or more until nicely golden brown, then add remaining ingredients except for zucchini and stir until mixed.

Press the 'keep warm' button, shut the instant pot with its lid in the sealed position, then press the 'manual' button, press '+/-' to set the cooking time to 8 minutes and cook at high-pressure setting; when the pressure builds in the pot, the cooking timer will start.

When the instant pot buzzes, press the 'keep warm' button, do a quick pressure release and open the lid.

Taste the soup to adjust seasoning, add zucchini noodles and toss until just mixed.

Ladle the soup into bowls and serve.

Nutrition:

Calories: 239;

Carbohydrates: 3g;

Protein: 29g;

Fat: 11g;

Sugar: 5g;

Sodium: 254mg;

Fiber: 1g

Broccoli Cheese Soup

Preparation Time: 10 minutes

Cooking Time: 12 minutes

Servings: 5

Ingredients:

2 tablespoons Butter, unsalted

2 tablespoons Minced garlic

3 cups Vegetable broth

6-ounce Broccoli florets

1 cup Monterey jack cheese, shredded

2 cups, and 2 tablespoons Sharp cheddar cheese, shredded

1 tablespoon Dijon mustard

½ teaspoon Paprika

⅛ Teaspoon Ground black pepper

1 cup Heavy whipping cream

¼ teaspoon Salt

1 teaspoon Xanthan gum

Directions:

Switch on the instant pot, add butter, press the 'sauté/simmer' button, wait until the butter melts and add garlic and cook for 1 minute or until fragrant.

Stir in broth, cook for 1 minute, then add broccoli florets and stir until mixed.

Press the 'keep warm' button, shut the instant pot with its lid in the sealed position, then press the 'manual' button, press '+/-' to set the cooking time to 10 minutes and cook at high-pressure setting; when the pressure builds in the pot, the cooking timer will start.

When the instant pot buzzes, press the 'keep warm' button, do quick pressure release and open the lid.

Add mustard, Monterey jack cheese, and 2 cups of cheddar cheese, season with black pepper and paprika and stir until cheese begins to melt.

Then pour in the cream, stir until well-incorporated and taste to adjust salt.

Take out ¾ cup of soup, add xanthan gum, stir well, then add into the soup in the instant pot and stir well until well combined.

Garnish soup with remaining cheddar cheese and serve.

Nutrition:

Calories: 276;

Carbohydrates: 5.1g;

Protein: 11.8g; Fat: 23.8g;

Sugar: 2.2g; Sodium: 509mg;

Fiber: 0g

Snacks and Sauces

Nutty spread Power Granola

Preparation time: 10 minutes

Cooking time: 5 minutes

Servings: 12 servings

Ingredients:

1 1/2 cups of almonds

1 1/2 cups of walnuts

1 cup destroyed coconut or almond flour

1/4 cup of sunflower seeds

1/3 cup of Swerve Sweetener

1/3 cup of vanilla whey protein powder

1/3 cup of nutty spread

1/4 cup of margarine

1/4 cup of water

Directions:

Preheat broiler to 300F and line a huge rimmed heating sheet with a paper material.

In a food processor, process almonds and walnuts until they look like coarse scraps with some bigger parts. Move to a large bowl and mix with destroyed coconut, sunflower seeds, sugar, and vanilla protein powder.

In a microwave-safe bowl, soften the nutty spread and margarine together.

Pour softened nutty spread blend over nut blend and mix well, stirring gently. Mix in water. Blend will cluster together.

Spread blend evenly on a prepared sheet and heat for 30 minutes. Take it out and let it cool.

Nutrition:

Calories: 338 kcal

Total Fat: 17g

Saturated Fat: 3.5g

Sodium: 80mg

Total Carbohydrates: 60g

Fiber: 8g

Total Sugars: 14g

Snickerdoodle Truffles

Preparation time: 10 minutes

Cooking time: 10 minutes

Servings: 4 servings

Ingredients:

2 cups of almond flour

1/2 cup of Swerve, Confectioners

1 tsp. of cream of tartar

1 tsp. of ground cinnamon

1/4 tsp. of salt

6 tbsps. Spread, softened

1 tsp. of vanilla concentrate

3 tbsps. Swerve, Granular

1 tsp. of ground cinnamon

Directions:

In a large bowl, whisk together the almond flour, Swerve, cream of tartar, cinnamon, and salt. Mix in dissolved spread and vanilla concentrate until the batter meets up. In the event that the mixture is too brittle to even think about squeezing together, add a tablespoon of water and mix together.

Scoop mixture out by the adjusted tablespoon and crush in your palm a couple of times to help in binding, at that point fold into a ball. Spot on a waxed paper sheet and rehash with residual batter.

In a shallow bowl, whisk together the Swerve and the cinnamon. Roll the truffles in the covering until all around secured.

Nutrition:

Calories: 121

Total Fat: 8.9g

Cholesterol: 0mg

Sodium: 201mg

Total Carbs: 5.8g

Fiber: 2.4g

Sugars: 0.2g

Protein: 4g

Pesto Zoodles

Preparation time: 10 minutes

Cooking time: 10 minutes

Servings: 4 servings

Ingredients:

2 cups of new basil leaves

1 garlic clove, crushed

1/3 cup of pine nuts

3 tablespoons of ground Parmesan cheddar

1/3 cup of extra-virgin olive oil, or a variant

Salt and newly ground dark pepper

1 tablespoon of extra-virgin olive oil

1 sweet onion daintily cut

4 zucchinis cut into noodles (utilizing a device like this)

Parmesan cheddar twists, for garnishing

Red-pepper pieces, for decorating (discretionary)

Directions:

Make the Pesto: In a food processor or blender, beat the basil, garlic, pine nuts, and ground Parmesan until coarsely slashed.

With the food processor running, include the olive oil gradually and blend until the pesto is thick like glue. Add progressively the olive oil varying to alter the consistency. Add pepper and salt.

Make the Zoodles: In a large sauté container, heat the oil over medium warmth. Include the onion and sauté until delicate, or for 4 to 5 minutes. Include the zucchini noodles and sauté until delicate, or for 4 to 5 minutes more.

Include the pesto and stir until the noodles are very much covered.

Serve warm, decorated with Parmesan twists and red-pepper pieces, if used to taste.

Nutrition:

Calories: 422

Total Fat: 36.3g

Cholesterol: 0mg

Sodium: 201mg

Total Carbs: 24.4g

Fiber: 3.9g

Sugars: 5g

Protein: 6.5g

Low Carb BBQ Sauce

Preparation time: 10 minutes

Cooking time: 5 minutes

Servings: 1-16 ounces

Ingredients:

1/4 cup of Lakanto Gold dark colored sugar substitute OR sugar of your choice

1/4 cup of apple juice vinegar

1/4 cup of white vinegar

1/2 cup of water

2 tablespoons of genuine spread

1 would tomato be able to glue

1 teaspoon of garlic powder

1 teaspoon of onion powder

1 teaspoon of dry yellow mustard

1 teaspoon of salt

1 teaspoon of cayenne pepper (discretionary)

1 teaspoon of fluid smoke (discretionary)

Directions:

If you like a thinner sauce, add more water until desired thickness is achieved.

If you like an increasingly acrid sauce, add more vinegar.

Go simple with the fluid smoke, a little is enough!

This formula is effectively versatile to various sugars. Utilizing a white sugar will bring about a sauce that is increasingly red in color.

The margarine makes a pleasant lustrous completion and makes the sauce to be on whatever you brush it on.

Nutrition:

Calories: 35

Total Fat: 0.4g

Cholesterol: 0mg

Sodium: 1198mg

Total Carbs: 5.9g

Fiber: 1.4g

Sugars: 3g

Protein: 1.3g

Tzatziki

Preparation time: 10 minutes

Cooking time: 0 minutes

Servings: 8 servings

Ingredients:

½ c shredded cucumber, drained

1 tsp. salt

1 T olive oil

1 T fresh mint, finely chopped

2 garlic cloves

1 c full-fat Greek yogurt

1 t lemon juice

Directions:

Place shredded cucumber on a strainer for an hour or squeeze out moisture through a cheesecloth.

Mix all ingredients in a medium bowl

Refrigerate.

Use as a vegetable dip, a dip for dehydrated vegetables, or a sauce for lamb, beef, or chicken. It is also a perfect accompaniment for fried summer squash.

Nutrition:

Calories: 79

Carbohydrates: 3g

Protein: 1g

Fat: 7g

Satay Sauce

Preparation time: 10 minutes

Cooking time: 15 minutes

Servings: 4 servings

Ingredients:

1 can (14 oz.) coconut cream (if you can't find coconut cream, coconut milk works well)

1 dry red pepper, seeds removed, chopped fine

1 clove garlic, minced

¼ cup gluten-free soy sauce

⅓ c natural unsweetened peanut butter

salt and pepper

Directions:

Place all ingredients in a small saucepan. Bring the mixture to a boil

Stir while heating to mix peanut butter with other ingredients as it melts.

After the mixture boils, turn down the heat to simmer on low heat for 5 to 10 minutes.

Remove from heat when the sauce is at the desired consistency. Adjust seasoning to taste.

This is a good sauce for chicken or turkey. Just add the sauce during the last minutes of baking or grilling. It can also be used as a dipping sauce.

Nutrition:

Calories: 312

Carbohydrates: 7g

Protein: 7g

Fat: 30g

Thousand Island Salad Dressing

Preparation time: 5 minutes

Cooking time: 5 minutes

Servings: 8 servings

Ingredients:

2 Tbs. olive oil

¼ c frozen spinach, thawed

2 T dried parsley

1 T dried dill

1 t onion powder

½ t salt

¼ t black pepper

1 c full-fat mayonnaise

¼ c full-fat sour cream

Directions:

Combine all ingredients in a small mixing bowl.

Nutrition:

Calories: 312

Carbohydrates: 2g

Protein: 1g

Fat: 34g

Hollandaise Sauce

Preparation time: 10 minutes

Cooking time: 15 minutes

Servings: 4 servings

Ingredients:

4 egg yolks

2 T lemon juice

1 ½ sticks of butter, melted

Salt and pepper

Directions:

Heat water to boil in a saucepan

Separate the eggs. Save the whites for another use.

Place the yolks in a heat-resistant bowl, either glass or stainless steel.

Carefully melt the butter in a saucepan without burning.

Place the bowl with the egg yolks over the simmering water to gently heat the eggs. Make sure the water is not touching the bottom of the bowl. The eggs need to be steamed, not cooked.

Add lemon juice to egg yolks.

Slowly stream the melted butter into the egg yolks while whisking. Start with a few drops of butter and then add a slow stream. Whisk the eggs the entire time until all the butter is added, and the sauce has thickened.

Season to taste with lemon juice, salt, and pepper; you can also add a dash of Tabasco sauce.

Serve over poached eggs or cooked vegetables.

Nutrition:

Calories: 566

Carbohydrates: 1g

Protein: 3g

Fat: 62g

Taco Flavored Cheddar Crisps

Preparation time: 5 minutes

Cooking time: 10 minutes

Servings: 6 servings

Ingredients:

¾ c sharp cheddar cheese, finely shredded

¼ c parmesan cheese, finely shredded

¼ t chili powder

¼ t ground cumin

Directions:

Preheat the oven to 400 degrees.

Line cookie sheet with parchment paper

In a bowl, toss all ingredients together until well mixed.

Make 12 piles of cheese parchment paper.

Press down the cheese into a thin layer of cheese.

Bake for 5 minutes until cheese if bubby.

Allow to cool on parchment paper.

When completely cool, peel the paper away from the crisps.

These are a good Keto substitute for chips. They are cheesy and crisp. Enjoy!

Nutrition:

Calories: 63

Fat: 5g

Sodium: 102mg

Total Carbs: 0.5g

Fiber: 0.1g

Sugars: 0.1g

Protein: 4g

Keto Seed Crispy Crackers

Preparation time: 10 minutes

Cooking time: 45 minutes

Servings: 30 servings of 1 cracker

Ingredients:

⅓ cup almond flour

⅓ cup sunflower seed kernels

⅓ cup pumpkin seed kernels

⅓ cup flaxseed

⅓ cup chia seeds

1 tbsp. ground psyllium husk powder

1 tsp. salt

¼ cup melted coconut oil

1 cup boiling water

Directions:

Preheat the oven to 300 degrees.

Stir all dry ingredients together in a medium-sized bowl until thoroughly mixed.

Add coconut oil and boiling water to dry ingredients and stir until all ingredients are mixed well.

On a flat surface, roll the dough between two pieces of parchment paper until approximately ⅛ inch thick.

Slide the dough, still between parchment papers onto a baking sheet.

Remove the top layer of parchment paper and place dough on a baking sheet into the oven.

Bake 40 minutes until golden brown.

Score the top of the dough into cracker sized pieces.

Leave in the oven to cool down.

When the big cracker is cool, break into pieces

These crackers can be stored in an airtight container after they are completely cool.

Nutrition:

Calories: 61

Carbohydrates: 1g

Protein: .2g

Fat: .6g

Dessert Recipes

Almond Cookies

Preparation Time: 10 minutes

Cooking Time: 20 minutes

Servings: 18

Ingredients

2 tbsp. Almond butter

1 tbsp. Coconut oil

¼ cup Coconut milk

2 tbsp. Sugar-free coconut syrup

2 large Eggs

½ tsp. Baking powder

½ tsp. Salt

2 tbsp. Granulated sugar substitute

1 ½ cup Sugar-free dried coconut

½ cup Flax meal

2 squares 90% dark chocolate

18 Almonds

Directions:

In a bowl, combine the coconut oil and almond butter and mix well.

Add the eggs, syrup, and coconut milk and mix until smooth.

Stir in the flax meal, dried coconut, sweetener, salt, and baking powder.

Roll the dough into 18 (1-inch) balls and place on a parchment covered cookie sheet.

Press lightly to make a dent on each ball.

Top with chopped chocolate (each cookie) and top with an almond.

Bake in a preheated 375F/190C oven until browned and slightly puffed, about 20 minutes.

Serve.

Nutrition:

Calories 114

Fat 11g

Carb 4g

Protein 3g

Pumpkin Pie Cupcakes

Preparation Time: 15 minutes

Cooking Time: 30 minutes

Servings: 6

Ingredients

3 Tbsp. Coconut flour

1 tsp. Pumpkin pie spice

¼ tsp. Baking powder

¼ tsp. Baking soda

Pinch salt

¾ cup Pumpkin puree

1/3 cup Swerve brown

¼ cup Heavy whipping cream

1 Egg

½ tsp. Vanilla

Directions:

Line 6 muffin cups with parchment paper and preheat the oven to 350F.

In a bowl, whisk together the salt, baking soda, baking powder, pumpkin pie spice, and coconut flour.

In another bowl, whisk egg, vanilla, cream, sweetener, and pumpkin puree until mixed. Whisk in dry ingredients.

Pour into the muffin cups and bake until just puffed and almost set, about 25 to 30 minutes.

Remove and cool.

Refrigerate for about 1 hour.

Top with whipped cream and serve.

Nutrition:

Calories: 70

Fat: 4.1g

Carb: 5.1g

Protein: 1.7g

Brownies

Preparation Time: 15 minutes

Cooking Time: 20 minutes

Servings: 16

Ingredients

½ cup, melted Butter

2/3 cup Swerve sweetener

3 Eggs

½ tsp. Vanilla extract

½ cup Almond flour

1/3 cup Cocoa powder

1 Tbsp. Gelatin

½ tsp. Baking powder

¼ tsp. Salt

¼ cup Water

1/3 cup Sugar-free chocolate chips

Directions:

Grease a (8 x 8-inch) baking pan and preheat the oven to 350F.

In a bowl, whisk together eggs, vanilla extract, sweetener, and butter.

Add the salt, baking powder, gelatin, cocoa powder, and flour and whisk until combined. Stir in the chocolate chips.

Fill the prepared baking pan with the batter.

Bake until center still a bit wet, but the edges are set, about 15 to 20 minutes.

Remove, cool, slice, and serve.

Nutrition:

Calories: 110

Fat: 9.5g

Carb: 3.6g

Protein: 3.1g

Ice Cream

Preparation Time: 15 minutes

Cooking Time: 30 minutes

Servings: 8

Ingredients

2 ½ cups, divided Heavy whipping cream

¼ cup Swerve brown

¼ cup Sugar substitute

2 Tbsp. Butter

1 ½ tsp. Maple extract

¼ tsp. Xanthan gum

1/3 cup Chopped walnuts

Directions:

In a saucepan, bring two sweeteners, and 1 ¼ cups of the whipping cream to a simmer. Lower heat and gently simmer for 30 minutes.

Remove from the heat and whisk in maple extract, and butter. Add the xanthan gum and whisk to mix well. Cool, and then place in the refrigerator for about 2 hours.

Beat the remaining whipping cream in a bowl until stiff peaks. Foil in chilled cream/maple until well combined. Stir in chopped walnuts.

Freeze until firm.

Serve.

Nutrition:

Calories: 318

Fat: 31.7g

Carb: 2.9g

Protein: 2.8g

Conclusion

Now that you are familiar with the Keto diet on many levels, you should feel confident in your ability to start your own Keto journey. This diet plan isn't going to hinder you or limit you, so do your best to keep this in mind as you begin changing your lifestyle and adjusting, you're eating habits. Packed with good fats and plenty of protein, your body is going to go through a transformation as it works to see these things as energy. Before you know it, your body will have an automatically accessible reserve that you can utilize at any time. Whether you need a boost of energy first thing in the morning or a second wind to keep you going throughout the day, this will already be inside of you.

As you take care of yourself through the next few years, you can feel great knowing that the Keto diet aligns with the anti-aging lifestyle that you seek. Not only does it keep you looking great and feeling younger, but it also acts as a preventative barrier from various ailments and conditions. The body tends to weaken as you age, but Keto helps to keep a shield up in front of it by giving you plenty of opportunities to burn energy and create muscle mass. Instead of taking the things that you need in order to feel great, Keto only takes what you have in abundance. This is how you will always end up feeling your best each day.

Arguably one of the best diets around, Keto keeps you feeling so great because you have many meal options! There is no shortage of delicious and filling meals that you can eat while you are on any of the Keto diet plans. You can even take this diet with you as you eat out at restaurants and at friends' houses. As long as you can remember the simple guidelines, you should have no problems staying on track with Keto. Cravings become almost non-existent as your body works to change the way it digests. Instead of relying on glucose in your bloodstream, your body switches focus, it begins using fat as soon as you reach the state of ketosis that you are aiming for. The best part is you do not have to do anything other than eating within your fat/protein/carb percentages. Your body will do the rest on its own.

Because this is a way that your body can properly function for long periods of time, Keto is proven to be more than a simple fad diet. Originating with a medical background for helping epilepsy patients, the Keto diet has been tried and tested for decades. Many successful studies align with the knowledge that Keto really works. Whether you are trying to be on the diet for a month or a year, both are just as healthy for you. Keto is an adjustment, but it is one that will continue benefiting you for as long as you are able to keep it up. If you are ready to feel great and look great from the inside out, you can begin your Keto journey with the confidence that it is truly going to make a difference in your life. The natural signs of aging and hormonal imbalances of being a woman are not enough to hold you back when you are actively participating in a balanced Keto diet.

Change your life today and enjoy the many benefits of a Keto diet.

CPSIA information can be obtained
at www.ICGtesting.com
Printed in the USA
LVHW011305221220
674886LV00001B/143

9 781914 092428